OWN YOUR BODY

GET THE BODY YOU WANT BY LEARNING HOW TO TAKE OWNERSHIP OF "YOU" TODAY!

DAVID ANTHONY

Outskirts Press, Inc.
http://www.outskirtspress.com

ISBN: 978-1-4787-4172-5

Outskirts Press and the "OP" logo are trademarks belonging to Outskirts Press, Inc.

PRINTED IN THE UNITED STATES OF AMERICA

outskirts press

TABLE OF CONTENTS

INTRODUCTION

Welcome to Own Your Body. I have written this book for both men and women. My main objective is to show you how to take ownership of your body through proper diet, and exercise, while at the same time tapping into your spiritual strength to achieve true health and fitness from the inside out.

Own Your Body is for the everyday person that wants to make a change and is seeking real advice. That person is you. By picking up this book named "Own Your Body" you have shown that you are seeking ownership of yourself, you are ready to take your body back and are ready to own up to achieving your goal of having and enjoying a healthier lifestyle.

In today's world of mass media and the social networking age, it is easy to get lost in so much information and opinions that are out there. Just what is real and what is not? What is simply an advertisement blog or commercial and what is a real person that has gotten real results? How do you know? There are so many viewpoints, it seems that for every good thing you read about, you can also find a negative thing on it as well. You don't know if the negative was just written by a paid blogger or if the good thing was written by the product manufacturer. With so much information especially about diet, fitness and natural health, so many websites trying to sell you something, it is understandable how a person can become overwhelmed and confused with what to do or who to listen to. We begin to overthink things many times, just plain giving up before we have even started. This may have happened with you as well. This is one reason my staff does not get commission and we accept no incentives to suggest certain products. We talk about what has been proven and what we know to be successful for the majority of our clients.

That is why I have chosen to write this book. I have spent the last several years in my nutrition center weeding out the good from the bad, what is real and what is just hype. And the most important part is who is really getting results from the products taken that I see first hand. It is not hype or hearsay, it is real results by real everyday people. I have opportunities every day to bring new products into our inventory and the salespeople come in daily offering deals, promotions to sell me products that are, many times, just repeats of what is already on the market with a new label and ad campaign. Just be observant. We simply will not bring a product onto our shelves until we make sure it is the right one, that it is true to its label claims, it's real and it works. I sort through all the thousands of products in the marketplace so you don't have to and we try to bring in the best possible.

You see, in today's market, with so many get rich schemes, some companies will just hire a spokes model or athlete to be pictured with the product, even though they have never even taken it long enough to present any true results. They just want you to buy it. Or the companies will post ads in the magazines and put fitness routines and diets that the average person with a job and any type of real schedule would never be able to follow. They know very well that you will buy the product and then blame yourself for not following through on taking it. This leads to the endless trials and false starts along with adding a shelf of products never finished that so many of you have. That is what leads to the term "roller coaster dieting."

The same is true with the fitness club industry as well; it will be packed in January and February for all the New Year's resolutions. Everyone is trying those new diets and workout programs that are not suited for them or their lifestyle and then by the true year after year tradition, fitness clubs will be half empty again by the end of March with as many as 70-80% of those people not sticking to working out and diets, simply giving up all because they started on the wrong path and were set up to fail by being given the wrong information. So then in another month they will go back and buy another product, and then another later, leading to the constant repeat of the endless dieters and the endless fitness routines. These make product manufacturer companies rich and at the same time leave you unhealthy and out of shape with frustration, depression, insecurity and less motivation than when you started. Don't get me wrong, many people make it; but they must step out of the typical consumer mold and find the store and products they can trust, a good trainer they can trust, the right information and proper mentor. Many times that proper mentor is standing right with you, encouraging faith in God which leads to faith in yourself. Believe, own it, and you will achieve it!

So who am I and how do I know? I started working in the fitness industry in 1985, over thirty years ago, and this is where I got my first experience in the fitness club environment. I since have become a nutritional entrepreneur and have opened and owned five different nutrition center locations and am the owner and co-founder of the Nature's Market & Fitness Nutrition Center in Orlando, Florida. I launched this with my business partner over twenty years ago. We have grown to be one of the oldest, highest volume, privately owned nutrition centers in Orlando, with 3rd and 4th family generations shopping us as we are known for quality products. We are also known for the knowledge, trustworthiness and help we give our customers. We have helped and literally counceled thousands of customers with their health related issues over the period of twenty years that we have been open, and there is very little that we have not seen or had experience in dealing with over the years.

Now at fifty plus years of age, I am a competitive bodybuilder and masters champion. I also hold triple certifications in personal training and nutrition. I am a Medical Exer-Therapist, specializing in training of persons with health related medical issues. I also have been involved in the formulation, production and distribution of nutritional supplements. We have several of our own exclusive, highly rated products for both men and women, from prostate health and testosterone boosting, to menopause, fat loss, arthritis, brain memory and cardiovascular health produced on our Nature's Market and Olympia Health lines. So when I talk to you about products, I know the industry, from the raw materials, to the manufacturing and distribution, to the consultation and the final results. Our products go through lab testing as most products in our store do, to assure you get the best quality at the best price. We truly are a results driven company. Never have we been a money driven company. It has always been about loving what we do and doing it well. The rest just comes with it and that is my advice to everyone when it comes to employment or owning a business, just do what you love.

I am a registered member of the National Physique Committee (N.P.C.) and the National Nutritional Foods Association (N.N.F.A.), both established and recognized as leaders in the fitness and natural health industry. I have sponsored the Orlando Muscle Classic and work very closely with several fitness clubs, personal training facilities, natural doctors including one on my staff. My store works with many athletic departments from the local schools, several nutritional and dietary organizations and even traditional doctors and chiropractors that send their patients in to us. The nutritional, natural health, traditional doctors and pharmaceutical industries can all work together if they try, and this will yield the best overall results for each person and a much healthier world. There is never failure in trying.

Always have a doctor that values nutrition as well as traditional medicine and that values the quality of life first.

I look forward to helping you learn how to take control of your body both on a physical and spiritual level. No matter how old you are, what your gender is, how much money you make, how much time you have, what religion you are, what health ailments you may have, we can for sure work together to put you on the right path to a better and healthier you. I am not a trainer of any of the big movie stars, but I am a trainer of common people just like you that want real results, of people who can't have a traveling chef and trainer 24/7, just desiring real information and real results for everyday people. It is time for the true information to be given from someone that has been around the real fitness and nutrition industry for many years.

Stay involved in your own health, seek your physician's advice and get regular check-ups and blood work. But also remember this is your body and you own the rights to it. So you can follow a balanced nutrition and fitness program to enhance your quality of life and not just rely on medications that are often over prescribed. Some things can be helped with just some lifestyle changes. But always work with your physician in doing so, and as with everything, find the right one and own your health.

A well known reverend once said, "All people are the same, some just have bigger dreams." Don't let anyone take your dreams and goals away from you. Claim your dreams as yours and own them!

Never forget that many great things all started as someone's dream. Believe in God, believe in yourself, and believe that you can achieve your goals, and you will. Own your fitness dream, start today!

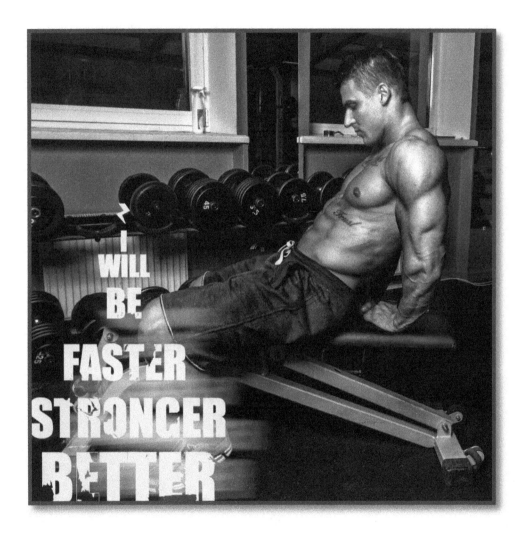

Let everyone you come in contact with

become a better person because of your meeting.

Bring improvement through encouragement.

Perform this exercise on someone today.

Remember to own your ability to encourage.

This world can and should be a better place

because of your time here.

Let it start with you.

Make a difference,

Be the difference!

CHAPTER ONE
OWNING YOUR BODY

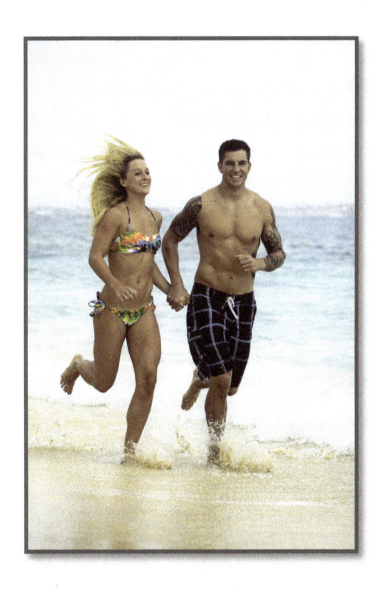

CHAPTER ONE
OWNING YOUR BODY

Do you own your body? We all just assume that we own our bodies, of course we do, right? Well, if you own it, then why can't you take control of it? We all see those perfect bodies walking by and many of you wonder just how they got in such good shape. Then we start to make ourselves feel better by saying, "Oh, it's their genetics," and so on, but in reality, it is the ownership they have of their bodies.

Your body works for you, that's its job. You are its employer, so you give the body the proper training and tools to get the job done, and it will. You own it, now take ownership of your body today and you will be making the best investment for your future. It's time for you to build your business, the business of a better body, the business of getting fit and healthy. It's time for you to OWN IT!

Who or what controls your day? Who or what owns so much of you that you have no time to exercise or follow a diet?

Who owns your time? You do, don't you? Or is it your television programs, your Facebook account, cell phone/texting, family obligations, cigarettes and alcohol, work, fast foods … the list can go on and on.

Take back the ownership of YOU and take control of your body, your eating habits, the management of your time, the work schedule you follow. Simply put, just take back what is yours; claim ownership of your life. You own it!

Basically this is about time management. Plan and organize your week in advance. You must plan to succeed. Not planning is just a plan to fail.

Who is controlling who? Is your life controlling you, or are you controlling your life? Many people these days are controlled by their computers or phones, even a website they favor. But shouldn't it be the other way around?

Stop allowing these outside distractions to keep you away from your goals. I am amazed sometimes that people take their cell phones into the gym and try talking on them during their workouts. You must give 100% concentration to your workouts, so leave the cell phone in the locker and don't let your bad habits ruin your workout and someone else's workout as well, remember to focus.

To be organized, you must plan your workout schedule and prepare your food in advance. Let's say you prepare your food on a Sunday and then store it in the refrigerator in Tupperware-like containers for easy access and freshness. As an example, bake chicken breasts, skinless, for each day of the week. Prepare a bowl of brown rice and some chopped vegetables. This kind of planning allows you to come home and simply pop the food in the microwave and have a nutritious dinner in five minutes, eliminating temptations to stop for fast food or cook something unhealthy. Plus the time you saved from not having to cook gives you thirty minutes that you can apply to a workout. Organization and proper planning are the key steps to a fit body and owning your schedule.

Being organized is a big part of time management. TV shows you enjoy can be recorded on DVR and watched anytime. You can limit your time on Facebook to every other day or no more than 20-30 minutes per day. You don't have to answer every cell phone call or text until you have time to do so, unless there is an emergency situation.

Take control and ownership of your body. Organization can be the key to your success in a diet and fitness routine. You must be serious and treat your body as a priority because without good health you cannot achieve anything else you need to do. The body must be respected. It is truly a miracle in itself. Be proud of who you are, big or small, fat or skinny, because you are a miracle. It is now time to take ownership of your body and who you are and fix it to be the best "YOU" that "YOU" can be.

I welcome you to your new level of ownership in YOU!

CHAPTER TWO
LOOKING GOOD IN TODAY'S WORLD

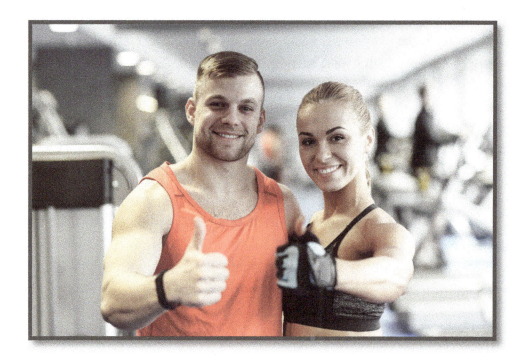

CHAPTER TWO
LOOKING GOOD
IN TODAY'S WORLD

There is more pressure today than ever before to look good, to look younger. Parents today want to look like their children's older sister or brother and not like their moms and dads.

In the work environment, older employees have to compete with the younger employees to look good, dress more appealing, and be in shape. Everyone fears they will be replaced based on looks and not performance. Image has become fifty percent of the job description in some cases.

Why? What has changed? Well, just about everything has changed. For starters, the retirement age is no longer sixty-two. People are expected to work until they are older now, so they need to stay serious and productive in the workplace or someone waiting in the wings, half the age, with a college degree, that can't find work and is willing to take a lesser salary might come take their job.

Next, the fast information and camera ready age we live in. You have to always be ready for someone to take your picture and place it on their Facebook or other sites on personal or business networks for millions of people to see.

Then there is television and magazine media constantly talking about fashion and what people are wearing or should be wearing. The commercials and ads for mini one-day facelifts, treatment for men's testosterone levels to stay younger. The hair and makeup products and the example of celebrities having perfect fashion and bodies along with the overabundance of infomercials on "get in shape quick" machines, diets, and routines In addition to that like it or not, all the dating sites are just a click away, ready to put temptation and doubt in a relationship right from home or office, a spouse can access and be on the lookout for the next best thing so easily today. It is important to stay looking good for your relationship as well, be the best you can be not only for yourself, but for your partner. I hate to mention it, but that is the truth and the divorce rate is fifty percent of all marriages, it is every married person's responsibility and anyone in a relationship, to still keep the spark alive in their relationship and look good for each other.

Yes, the pressure today is very high to be at your best and to stay looking as young as possible for as long as possible. My grandparents certainly did not look like the grandparents of today.

But you must remember that quick fixes like liposuction or bariatric bypass surgery to lose weight are just that — quick fixes. You must change your lifestyle or you will be right back where you started in one to three years. Take ownership of your body and make this a new way of life, using these quick fixes strictly in the case of health risk situations only or as jump starts for a real lifestyle change that you will stick with for the rest of your life.

I have personally seen clients in my counseling that have gone on these crash diets and undergone medical procedures for weight loss, thinking it was going to change their lives and everything that was wrong in life. However, after being overweight for a long time, some people start to use their weight problem as an excuse for everything that goes wrong in their lives. They find that once they lose the weight, some of those problems are still there. Then they get depressed and eat their way back to being overweight.

Being overweight is never an excuse for being lazy. Look at Governor Chris Christie of New Jersey. He is overweight but he never let it hold him back from his success. So when someone like him loses weight, they are more likely to be truly happy since they did not base their life on their size. They owned it and made it work for them. They took control from the inside first and now they are a perfect candidate to lose the weight for a true transformation on the outside. He also shows that just because someone is overweight, it does not have to limit their level of success. I was actually told to pull this part out in the book layout because of the bridge scandal in New Jersey. I thought that was interesting since the scandal has nothing to do with his weight, and I am an independent so I do not support any particular party. I have been in both parties and now I have learned to judge my vote on the individual, not the party. Politicians should have term limits of twelve years and campaign finance reform where they have to spend the same amounts of money to run and keep it to issues and not fancy commercials slinging mud at the other candidate. Then we will have more control of the people representing us in Washington again. But as long as they need big money to keep running campaigns, then their votes can be bought by big corporations and the American people lose out including the supplement industry since the pharmaceutical industry puts pressure on the votes of our elected officials to vote against nutritional supplements, which led to some very good ones being taken off the market. I did not worry about adding a politician into this chapter who is a good example of what an overweight person can still accomplish and still how much ridicule he can get from other grown adults on television. It's like some people are still in grade school with name calling and making fun of people's bodies. This is really something that we need to get past in our nation. Good people come in all shapes and sizes; we must all accept this and then we must all help each other to do and be better and healthier, but making fun of one another is not the answer, encouragement is.

So my advice is to be secure with who you are and be the best that you can be for your body type. Do not count on the loss of weight or the gaining of muscle to be used as a way to fix all your problems. Use them as stepping stones for a true lifestyle change. Fitness is and should be a way of life, something that you just do without thinking too much about it. Fitness needs to become a part of you like taking a shower, brushing your teeth, etc. You never hear anyone say, "Oh, I can't find time to brush my teeth." Right? (at least we hope not!) It just becomes a part of what is expected to be done, and that is what your fitness and nutrition goals need to be: a second nature, part of your routine, a true part of your life. When you get to that point, then you have taken ownership of your body.

You must change your mind set to stop thinking of a fitness routine or diet plan as work. If you're doing the proper exercise routine, you will actually get energy from your workout due to the blood and oxygen getting into your muscles and the blood flow circulation throughout the body. Plus it will raise your endorphins, putting you in a better mood and relieving stress. As far as a diet plan goes, well, you will be eating more frequently than ever before with small portions while losing weight at the same time, so there is no starvation going on. Taking ownership of your body is the best decision you can make for your quality of life, your loved ones, and your productivity at work. Plus, becoming a good example of achieving a true lifestyle change can be a positive influence and inspiration to other people in your life.

CHAPTER THREE
BALANCED

Balanced — Wow, what a word, so simple yet with so much power. But what does it really mean?

Webster's dictionary defines balanced several ways, but three stand out. The first defines balance as "harmonious proportion of elements," the second defines balance as "bodily or mental stability," and the third defines it as "to equalize" and "keep a state of equilibrium."

Life must have balance or it becomes lopsided. If you're in a boat and everyone moves to one side, the boat will tip and start to take on water. Life is the same way and so is your fitness and nutrition program. They must have a balance or it simply won't float.

Being balanced as we age means finally knowing what is important in life, recognizing what things to sweat and what things to let go of and not worry about. More isn't always better.

We must always take a look to see what is out of balance in our lives and what is stealing our time: our peace time, our fitness time, our family time, our diet time, our prayer time. Then we must center ourselves, take back the ownership of our lives, and regroup to properly prioritize the way we live. You will see a huge difference by taking the time to take back the ownership and control that leads to a true balanced you.

The importance of being balanced in your daily life leads to the control you need to take ownership of your fitness life.

The word balanced, I think, is one of the most important words in life. Having a good and happy life, while at the same time accomplishing your goals, means having a balance to go about your fitness lifestyle change.

Stop putting pressure on yourself to go so overboard in one or two areas of your life while at the same time letting other important areas go unattended.

Control and time management over your life is a must. It is better to accomplish a couple solid goals rather than have ten unfinished goals that never go anywhere. Less is more in many instances. Do you need to belong to every club? Attend every social? Does your child need to play every sport even though he is only good at one or two and should focus where his talents better serve him? Do you really need to meet the other people from work three nights a week after work? Can't it just be once every couple weeks? Do you really need two hours on social media sites nightly? Can't it be thirty minutes? Do you really need to cook every night? As I mentioned earlier, can't you prepare meals on your day off for the whole week and eat throughout the week from whatever you prepared in advance for 5 days. This can save 30 minutes to a hour per night that equals 5 hours a week, or 20 hours a month just to make dinner, (even if you spend half that time, equaling 10 hours per month). There is your workout time. My point is that there is always time that can be made to allow your workout in and to have less stress in your life.

Balanced — You can always have too much of something and too much is not good. Life is a balance and balance will have you happier and more fulfilled. You can have too much exercise, too much dieting, too much TV, too much working out, too much sex, and even too much religion. I say too much religion, but not too much faith in God or love for Him. Too much religion would be the meaning of too much structured opinion of the church and not enough actual living of the Word of God, being so wrapped up in the ritual that you may forget the importance of the personal relationship with God that is the true strength of your soul and the love that we are to have for one another.

Balanced in your relationship — This is big because a relationship can be lost in the mix of being busy and not allowing time for your relationship. You must take the time to keep things fresh and not get into a routine of habit. Do not feel guilty if you have kids and need an hour alone for your relationship. This hour of space together will strengthen the whole family unit. Don't forget why you fell in love with each other. Have someone watch the kids for date night, consider summer church camps for a week for the kids, giving you and your other half renewal time together. This could really make the difference between a couple that stays together and one that parts ways. I have had friends that have gotten married, then became lazy and stopped the gym, gained weight, became a different person than their spouse originally married and then wondered why they had problems. Be true to who you are, and be the best for you and your partner.

Balanced in your fitness — A little time can go a long way. It's about consistency and it does not mean two to three hours a day at the gym, thirty to sixty minutes, 3-4 days per week is fine, as long as you stay with it and watch the diet along with the fitness routine. Be the best that your body can be for your shape, and never blame it on the time because you can make time.

Balance in diet — Means following a good diet, the five to six small meals per day six days per week, but that doesn't mean if there is a special occasion you can't have a cheat meal. We must use common sense and remember if you decide to go to dinner with friends don't put the whole table through your menu diet drama. Never ask the calories to the server. Use common sense, order the chicken or fish, a vegetable, and salad. Don't involve the whole table since it makes people uncomfortable regarding what they might want to order and it puts you on stage with your diet, and it should not be about you. This is a way of life, again like brushing your teeth. Make it simple and non painful. If all else fails then drink a large glass of water before your meals and start with a green salad with vinegar and oil first to fill you up before the main meal comes and at home use smaller plates, tall skinny glasses for beverages, be all about portion control, give the illusion to your eye that the plate and glass are full, but in reality there is less food. Find ways that work for you and your family, they won't even know but will start to see the results. Find the ways to be balanced!

Balanced also means not to go from doing no exercise at all, to doing a maximum hard workout routine immediately that will leave you sore, fatigued, take up too much of your time and be too hard for you to follow and keep up, which would then give you the excuse that you tried and it just wasn't for you and that working out isn't for you. Do not try this excuse, start slow; even just two days a week while at the same time changing your diet, then when ready move up to three days a week. Starting two days a week can be as simple as walking, taking a jazzercise class or anything that keeps you moving and starts to train your mind and body, allowing you to be doing something active at that time of the day. Then build off of it and progress into a workout schedule and routine by adding more each time. Keep a balance, make the commitment to really do something for your body this time, the most expensive item you own is your health, handle it like the special jewel it is, there is not another like it. Owning the balance in your life that allows you to workout is the best exercise of all.

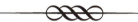

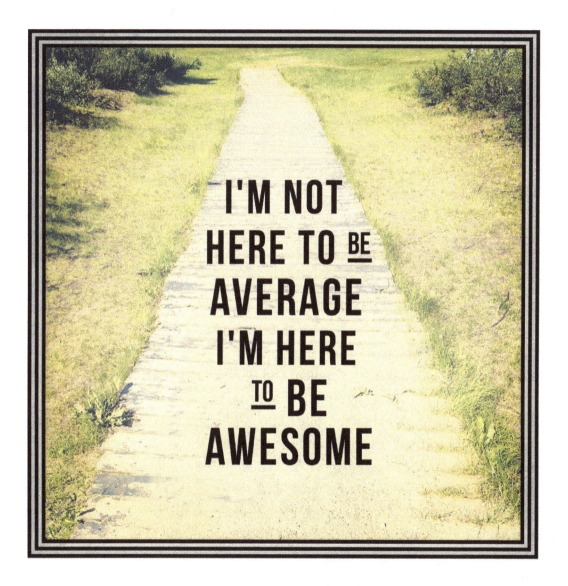

I'M NOT HERE TO BE AVERAGE I'M HERE TO BE AWESOME

CHAPTER FOUR
WHAT'S GENETICS GOT TO DO WITH IT?

Each one of us holds our own DNA profile. It's like a roadmap of who we are. But does it have anything to do with how fit we are?

We all hear people saying that they don't have the genetics to do this or that. Well, that might be true if it is someone 5'4" tall trying out for a spot on the NBA, but it does not have anything to do with physical fitness and the type of fit body you can achieve by a good consistent diet and exercise program.

Everyone inherits certain traits from their parents, like eye color and hair color, but according to the research of scientists labeled "epigenetic," they discovered our genes are approximately only 15 percent of our total genetics that we get from our parents, and the other 85 percent, labeled "epigenome," are proteins that form your DNA's profile and pattern. These proteins are working with the environment around you, your lifestyle choices. A study done by Dr. Martin in Oakland shows how it is possible to change the effect of one's own DNA and that of their children and grandchildren simply by leading a good diet and fitness lifestyle. There are studies that show how the effect of our own DNA changes to adapt to our environment and those changes become part of our DNA that gets passed along to our children and grandchildren.

Dr. Frank Lipman explained that while each of us inherit our own unique, hardwired, unchangeable version of the genetic code, epigenetic factors such as lifestyle and diet can significantly change what our genes do, especially where fitness is concerned.

In an article by Dr. Al Sears, he wrote that you can "talk" to your genes through lifestyle changes that can improve your health and possibly prevent disease in some cases, even if it runs in your family. He states that by taking the following vitamins, your body will start to modify and improve its genetic code.

Vitamins E (100 IUs), C (2000 mg), and A (5,000 IUs) normalize cell division. In just moderate doses some believe this can help prevent certain family related health problems. Vitamins B12 (1000 mcg), folic acid (500-1000 mcg), B-6 (20-50 mg), and

Betaine (500-1000 mg) all help to detox your bad genes, allowing for proper genetic code signaling and output.

So for some people to say, "It's the genetics," that just isn't so. You can stop that negative genetic effect by implementing change today. You have a choice to make and lead a healthy lifestyle. This can improve your overall health and appearance with a true lifestyle change that just might have an effect on your children and your children's children. Wow! What you do today can have lasting effects on generations to come. So start today in a new direction, not only for yourself, but for your family's future generations to come. There is much research being done on this topic, so look into this further if your family has a history of illness and start working to stop the bad genetic code link in your family genes, especially with your children.

The decisions you make and the actions you take today by taking ownership of your body for your outward physical fitness and internal health will have positive effects for years to come.

So what does genetics have to do with it? Well, as far as you getting into the best shape of your life and improving your overall health and lifestyle, nothing. You control the ownership of your fitness and health, not your genetics. You decide when you're going to work out and what you're going to eat, not your genetics. So the breaking of the "genetic code" for fitness is simple: Just get off your butt and do it!

Basically, the biggest point that I am trying to make with you is to let you know that regardless of your current body, large or small, doesn't matter, whatever it is, it can be better and that is a fact. Your genetics does not drive the car through the fast food drive thru or push the cart in the grocery store aisles, you do that. So each day you can do better than the day before. You can be a better you.

Don't let yourself say things like, "well the fat gene runs in my family and there is nothing I can do about it, I will never be thin, so I mine as well eat what I want to eat, It's my genetics, it's not my fault." You are in control of your thoughts and actions.

I even hear similar comments from guys in the gym that have not trained legs properly, or neglected them for a long period of time just to do upper body which is always what the guys want first, a big chest and arms, and they will say they don't have the genetics for big legs or calves, well this is just not true. Or they come up to me and say I have good genetics and that is how I have good legs and calves, and I will tell them no, I have good legs and calves from hard work, squatting, calf raises ect...and that I do not have great genetics, I had skinny stick legs and a mother over 300lbs, my "Genetics " did not get me this physique, it was hard training, diet and consistency with a goal in mind to achieve and work towards. You own your genetics, don't let them own you!

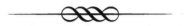

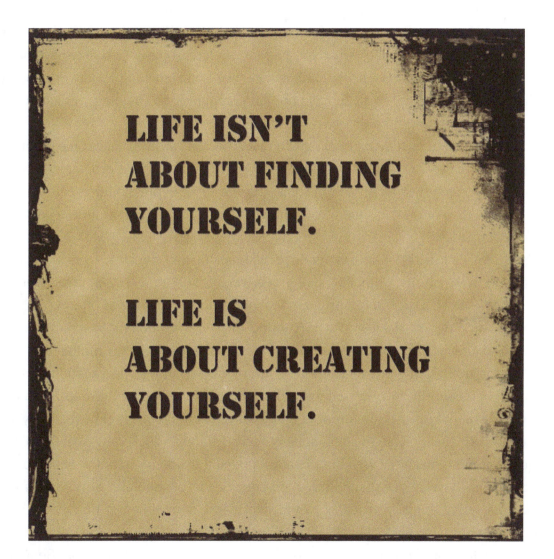

LIFE ISN'T
ABOUT FINDING
YOURSELF.

LIFE IS
ABOUT CREATING
YOURSELF.

CHAPTER FIVE
A BODY TRANSFORMATION

Most of you have tried various diets and nutrition programs that haven't worked for you. Some of you may have gotten good results from some diet and exercise programs, but you may have gained back what you had lost. In fact, some of you may have never tried any programs, and have never had the incentive to do anything about your bodies. Well, the time has come, and you have my full commitment to helping you get on the right track to a healthy and fit lifestyle.

I spend much of my day counseling frustrated men and women that come to me for advice because they are unable to tackle their weight loss and fitness programs. This has caused them much frustration, and in some cases, a silent depression that eats away at their insides. This also affects them at home with their families and at times even their work performance.

You see, I have first hand experience with all of this because I grew up in a household in which my mother was very overweight. She tried several diets over the years, then entered a special test program that one of the hospitals was offering. During that one-year program, she lost over 150 pounds. This was an incredible achievement. I remember our whole family beaming with pride. For the first time, my mother was able to shop for clothes, attend social events with my father, and go on vacation without being embarrassed to have her picture taken. I too was proud of her and no longer had to fear other kids making fun of her, as young children tend to do when they see someone very overweight. You see, society tends to always look only skin deep and forgets that there may very well be a beautiful person inside of an out of shape body. Unfortunately, your out of shape body then becomes a "prison cell," and it holds you back from doing things you really would like to do. Sometimes, it may hold those people closest to you back as well. Remember to lend your help, not the critical bully type words that can flow from one's mouth at a person that is out of shape. Be a part of the solution, not a part of the problem.

Growing up in this type of environment is what drew my interest into the fitness and nutrition industry. I still recall the first picture I saw of Arnold Schwarzenegger as Mr.

Universe when he was new in the Unites States, well before his Mr. Olympia win. I was about twelve years old at the time, I was awed at his physique as many were. It inspired me to get into a good fitness and nutrition program, and also to become goal oriented so that I could stick with it. I remember ordering my first body building program from an advertisement I found in the back of a comic book. It's a much different fitness world now. Back then I could only get a fitness magazine every six months called Iron Man and there were only two choices of protein powder at the health food store, They both tasted horrible and I had to hold my nose to drink them, but I kept the focus on my long term goal and not on the taste of the moment. Times have really changed in today's world, making it much easier to become fit in many ways do to everything we have at out finger tips now to help.

My goals also made me want to help others in their suffering. I knew the beauty of seeing someone "blossom" after they'd lost weight or as they strived to lose fat or build muscle. It's a great feeling to put on a pair of shorts and a tank top, or a bathing suit, and be comfortable with your body. I remember after a lot of heavy working out and the building of my physique, I was able to finally feel confident at the beach or pool. You see, what some people do not realize is that people that are very thin and can't gain weight also go through a similar frustration, only with the opposite needs. Either situation can become very serious to one's well-being. Also, remember to check with your physician. In some cases, you may have a thyroid disorder or sugar problems, for which your doctor can prescribe medication or some other alternative solution; however, you will still need to diet and exercise which in itself may take care of the problem.

I myself have always struggled with a "sweet tooth." Being Italian, I was used to such good cooking. But self control and discipline is what it is all about. Keep your eye on the end result and not on the moment of weakness or temptation.

Being Catholic and of Christian faith, I was always taught that during the forty days of Lent, I would give up my favorite food for the Lord, not being able to touch it again until Easter Sunday. (My father did this every year). This was an incredible living experience for me because I found that when I gave it up for the Lord, even the biggest, best dessert could be sitting right in front of me, and I wouldn't touch it. In fact, I loved the temptation because I always believed it was the devil trying to tempt me and I could show him time and again that the Lord would win, and not his temptation. In fact, when it came to the day I could finally eat the pastry, I didn't even really want it. I found I didn't really miss it as much as I once thought I did. You see, it's really the sugar that you're craving and not the sweets. Both sugar and salt can be addictive, just like a drug can be. You can also find substitutions for some of the things you like and slowly remove yourself from them, such as substituting ice cream or other desserts after dinner with fat-free/sugar-free yogurt cups. Keep chopped carrot and celery sticks as munchies. Take up some hobbies that will keep you busy instead of watching TV all night long. Only watch the shows you really like and start being productive in other areas of your life. Start planning on making a difference in your life and not just sitting in front of the television wasting precious time. Keeping busy and occupied is a great part of any diet and fitness routine.

If God were to call you home today, what would be said about your accomplishments tomorrow? What difference would you have made by being here? If you do not have an answer to these questions, then it is time to get busy. Volunteer to help people within your community. Do something that will be your legacy. God put us all here for a reason. He doesn't make mistakes. He didn't place you in your particular city or state surrounded by the family and friends you're with by accident. You've been placed where you are because He needs you to learn and grow within that particular environment. What you do with your situation is up to you because we were born with a thing God chose to give us called "self will." He leaves the final decisions up to us. We can all complain about what did or did not happen in our lives from the time we were growing up to even our current adulthood. It will not change the fact that God wanted us where we were to learn and grow. What we've done with it has been up to us on an individual basis. We must always see the cup as half full in all situations and focus on the good, even in the worst of times there is still good to be found. Some of us have done nothing but put blame on someone else or individual circumstances that surrounded them and there is no one to blame and no excuses except lack of focus and lack of faith and discipline. Pray for guidance and God will give it to you. The time is now, so let's do it. Trust in God and He will help guide you to taking ownership of your body.

If you haven't finished what you've started previously with your diet and fitness programs and other matters in your life, it's because you chose not to totally own it. Own your legacy, own your dreams, take ownership of your life. You can't remodel the house if you only rent it, so own it and get ready to remodel yourself today. He strengthens us in our weakness, and He steps in for us when we need Him to. He's an awesome God! He can when you can't.

In the following pages, you will find a schedule of step by step routine instructions. It will turn your lifestyle into a picture of health, happiness, and self-confidence from the inside out.

Most people do not realize that two of life's least time consuming activities will have the longest lasting positive results on their lives. These are prayer and working out, building the inner and outer self. Once you experience these two most important building blocks and link them together, then I know there will be no turning back. You'll be well on your way to achieving the best possible body for yourself.

God has blessed us with a miraculous body. It was formed in His image. It's the answer to our eternal life. Just look at the make up of the internal organs, along with our sense of touch, of smell, our feeling of love, the ability to reproduce, and the magnificent capability of the brain. Add to that the awesome inner soul that has a direct connection with our Heavenly Father, our Creator, to live on for all of eternity.

So many people take the body for granted. Always expecting it to be working the same at age fifty as it did at twenty-five years of age. That's not the case. It takes a thing called "Preventative Maintenance." just as you would perform preventative maintenance on your car or the air conditioning unit of your home, so it will not break down later. It is the same thing with our bodies.

Well, my friends, it's time for your body to have its "oil" changed, and to be put on a regular maintenance schedule. It's time to stop putting off owning up to the responsibility of your health. Do not let other things take ownership of you. Stay in control of your body, your health, your life. This is not being selfish or self centered. It's about taking care of your health for a true quality of life that will keep you here with your loved ones for many years to come. By owning your body today and letting it be the foundation pillar of so many great things that you will build upon, your health is your true physical foundation to a better you.

You are "one of a kind," you are priceless. Handle yourself with the care you deserve. You are a precious jewel in the crown of life. You are more than a millionaire; you are you, and that is special.

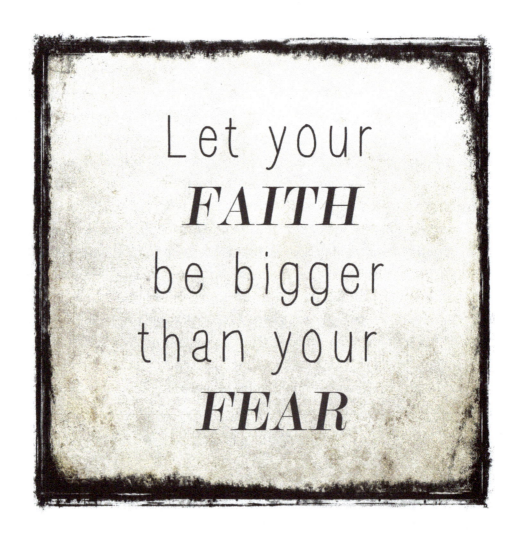

Let your **FAITH** be bigger than your **FEAR**

CHAPTER SIX
TAKING THE FITNESS CHALLENGE AT ANY AGE.

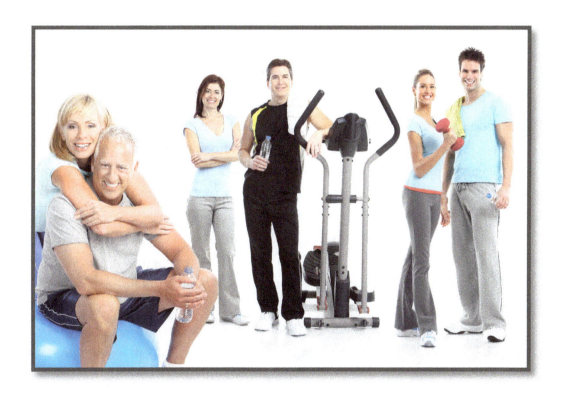

CHAPTER SIX
TAKING THE FITNESS CHALLENGE AT ANY AGE

Owning your fitness challenge at any age is a task that can and should be tried and is a very achievable and realistic goal when done right.

Many of us do not realize we have been trained to take a challenge since we were infants. So there is nothing new about taking the challenge of a new diet and/or workout routine.

The body has memory, it understands and adapts if we give it the right chance and time to do so. The body and mind understand a challenge because it has be trained to be challenged since early on.

The problem usually is that most people fear a challenge simply because they fear failing and do not understand that our body is ready and capable of achieving success if you just give it the tools to do so and do not fear getting out of your comfort level.

Yes, it is true, many of us have been trained for a challenge from our first steps, our first words, the first day of school, learning to read and write, learning the ABC's, our first ball toss, our first bike ride, solving your first math problem, making your bed for the first time, the first time you drove and so on... We complete challenges every day without even thinking about it and we conquer them and move onto the next and conquer again and so on, your diet and fitness routine is the same thing. Conquer it just like you have conquered so many other things in life.

A challenge is defined as "any thing that calls for a special effort." Make that special effort and take your challenge once again; you can and will do it. Remember that key word "effort." Yes, you will need to maybe go to bed earlier or wake up earlier. We all expect and want to see our home pro sports teams win, be it in football, baseball, basketball and now soccer, but don't you expect them to be making an effort to train and put the time in to get the team and fans to the finish line? Of course you do, you expect a special effort and if one of the team players was never at practice and getting out of shape, you would expect them to fire him, right? But when it comes to people trying to get into fitness and the body they want, they seem to look for a quick fix instead of wanting to put the effort in, that same effort you would expect from anyone that would be getting good results. Effort and discipline, you know what it is, you have had it before, you have enforced it before with teammates, or your children or friends, but now you have lost the focus and need to get back to understanding the simple fact that getting in shape requires you to make an effort! If you don't wash the clothes and keep putting them in a big pile, they eventually build a mound, and you run out of clothes and they are not going to wash themselves. You need to make the effort to do so and clean up the mess. It is the same with your body. If you don't get rid of the fat it will keep piling up into a big mound and it won't take care of itself, you have to clean it up. My point is, start to treat getting into shape whether it be fat loss, muscle gain or both, as any other household chore you do. It just needs to be done so do it.

Back when we were infants and then on to young adults, we never put so much thought into things we were challenged by, we just did them and never considered all the different angles. This calls for that same way of thinking, just do it: start your diet and fitness routine and don't over think it, don't give yourself excuses or ways out. It is never too late to challenge yourself to being better each day, and that is all it needs to be, baby steps. We learned this already early in life, as I said previously, it is the same now, take an additional step each day and soon you will be walking and then running to the finish line with your diet and fitness goals.

It is beneficial for all of us to be ready for a challenge at any age and in all areas of life. This competitive nature is who we are as a people and it dates back to our ancestry in all nations. This is how we got the drive for the Olympic spirit, for all nations to come together to take a challenge and share in their competitive edge. It does not matter where they are from, the entire world population understands competition and a challenge. They understand that they must try their best to push and max out their potential, and it is not always about winning. Much of it is about the journey and the challenge that gets you to that point to even be in the position of a possible win. That in itself is a great personal achievement, knowing the focus, hard work and sacrifice it takes, but the great reward it brings. Competition can really change a life and make you reach to new levels. I myself learned so much by competing and just how dedicated and strong I could be when faced with the challenge. But it is best taken one day at a time. I encourage everyone to get involved in some type of competition to challenge yourself, maybe it is a community walk for Cancer, or a bike ride, whatever you choose, even one of the state offered N.P.C. fitness or bodybuilding contests or a local sport team. These can be wonderful tools to teach you to reach new levels in challenging yourself. It will make you stronger for all areas of your life and really help you in your diet and fitness goals.

Competitions are challenges that push you to do better each time you participate, which then becomes the challenge of doing and getting better each time. This competitive edge in each of us just needs to be recognized and tapped into. You must find this inner strength and tap into it and then use it to achieve the physique and level of fitness that you desire. You will feel a level of self accomplishment that you have never felt before. This will help you in all areas of your life, including self respect and self love. You know the saying you must love yourself before you can love someone else. That is true in both love and respect for yourself. The happier you feel, the more you will accomplish and the more people you will begin to influence by your ambitious goals and self discipline.

In the past it was believed 30's was old, then 40's and then 50's. With each decade the bar keeps getting moved to the point now that even sixty can be the new fifty and fifty the new forty. As we advance with our nutrition and fitness awareness and have really started to watch what we eat and demand better choices at the grocery store and restaurants, along with the well known fact that we need to keep active and do some form of exercise, the results are amazing simply because we are becoming a younger looking nation. Most people truly do look better than their parents and grandparents did at the same age. Taking the challenge to look better and to hang onto youth and, most importantly, the quality of life, means a more active and productive senior crowd, helping keep those older folks we hold dear to our hearts around for a bit longer and with a quality of life and non-dependency on others, which is very important to anyone. We all want to keep our self respect and not be a burden on any one of our family members. Thinking ahead is important, start building yourself now so later in life you have the quality of life that you well deserve.

You must come to terms with the fact that there is no perfection, there is no perfect person. You have to realize that you are looking to improve your body, but you will still be you, just a better form of you. Just because you can't wear a size small slacks, doesn't mean you can't look great in a size medium. Do not let silly insecurities hold you back. People come in all shapes and sizes and anyone can still look great just by making some realistic improvements at first and then trying to do a little more each time. Before you know it, you will have made a body transformation and a true lifestyle change, and it all started with taking a small first step to your fitness challenge. You can't finish if you don't start. So take the challenge today.

You always want to keep learning and growing, this keeps you motivated to always be ready for the next challenge life may throw your way. As with myself, for over twenty years now I have helped people with their fitness goals and have prepared many for competitions, but I can tell you first hand that when I started competing, it was far different than doing it from the side lines. Competing was a true challenge and many times I thought I could easily wait and not do this particular contest and save it for another time, but I didn't. I kept my word to myself and to those I told, and one important thing is to obligate yourself to complete a challenge by telling others. Then you will have even more reason to get it done and to stick with it and see it through. No matter how much I thought I knew about competing and the preparations for it, it is totally different when you have to go through it yourself. It is a true challenge and growth experience.

It takes a major effort every day, in fact every minute of every day, but it is well worth it. You keep doing what you normally do schedule wise and you just adjust and adapt your eating, training, practice and so on around it. Still keep a balance between everyday life and your competing if you choose to ever do it. Involving the kids can be fun for the whole family. One of the trainers I hired to prep me for my posing routine had children and they loved watching me practice and then loved even more getting to come to the competition to see the routine finished. If you can't find time because of the kids, then make the kids a part of it too. It serves as a great example to them of what you can do and what they can do too. It is much better for your children to see you competing than smoking and drinking, so you will be doing this for them as well. You are teaching them to be the best that they can be and to strive for taking their body to the peak level of performance.

I remember traveling up to north Florida and getting to the hotel the night before the competition where all the tanned competitors would be signed in and weighed, everyone was entering the room, and all of us were discreetly trying to look at who was competing against us. Every time we saw a good physique we'd all feel the pressure and hope they were not in our division. It is funny but everyone does this; it can make you really start to stress because some people you may think look better, but in the judging you can score higher with things like better definition, more muscle balance and so on. No one really knows what the out come will be for sure until it is announced. This first competition was great, everyone was friendly and helpful and many of us were competing for the first time. I encourage trying for smaller local shows first and then working up. I can tell you when they first call your class out onto stage and you are standing there with a spot light and judges looking up at you, it can be a nerve stimulating situation. Then when they are calling for you to do quarter turns and mandatory poses and you're trying to listen to them and at the same time trying to remember what you were taught and practiced and still smile too, well it is something to go through. But even so, I do not mind the prejudging, which is really the contest and when it is all decided except for the overall competition. The hard part is the individual posing routine when it is only you on stage that night with a full audience and judges. The thing I have learned is to just go with it. If there is a mistake, don't let it throw you off. I had hesitations the first time I did a posing routine on stage, but then the following competitions I got better and then better to the point of taking the overall masters class on the last competition I did. The thing about it is that it makes you want to go back and keep getting better because each time you know you could have done something different and with each experience you grow and learn. If you do anything that makes you grow and learn, then it has been worth the time and effort. At the end of the day the judges are judging each person on achieving their own best possible physique and balance for their own body and it really was not about who you are standing next to on stage, the winner is the person that best prepared their own body to be in the proper balance and conditioning, it is not about who is better, it is about if you have met your own challenge.

We have awesome amazing bodies that are capable of so much physically, make sure you keep your body challenged. I had wanted to compete in bodybuilding since I was a teenager. It took me many years to actually make it happen, but it taught me that it is never too late to go after your dreams!

Remember FOCUS! FOCUS! FOCUS! Keeping focused by not allowing distraction is so important. Distraction is the weapon of defeat. It keeps you from obtaining your goals and your work, your relationships, your diet and so on. Remember to stay focused on the workout, not where you're going to do it at, just do it. Stay focused on your diet, not all the choices you have that confuse you, just do it. The main focus needs to be on your main goal of fitness and not distracted by all the other stuff that divides us and separates us. We shouldn't turn one side up against the other with who is right and wrong, whose supplements work and whose doesn't, what the internet article says versus what your trainer said. Whose workout routine works and so on. Don't get wrapped up in all that distraction, just focus on the main goal. There is room for many different opinions and ways of doing things; pick what you feel is right for you and try it. I tend to be a "back to the basics" type of guy with my clients and my own training. They are proven methods that have worked for many years and will always be reliable for anyone that sticks with them. Activity is the key to youth and a sound mind and body, so stay challenged to be active in your life, and your body will reward you with the quality of life that you are well deserving of. Own your challenge today.

CHAPTER SEVEN
FITNESS BY FAITH

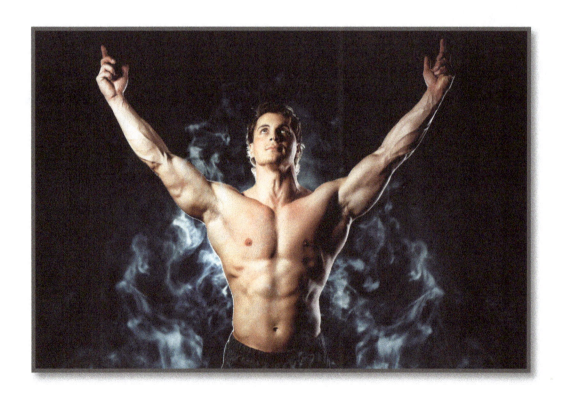

CHAPTER SEVEN
FITNESS BY FAITH

Own Your Faith

When you pray, ask God for the Holy Spirit to descend

upon you and help you achieve the willpower you need

to stick to this nutritional fitness program.

If you do this in the name of the Lord with Him

as your true spiritual personal trainer, then you

cannot fail! God does not fail and He will give you

the willpower and dedication you need to get

great results with this program,

but remember you have to trust in and believe in the

Lord's helping hand and not doubt Him and His help

and guidance in your fitness goals.

See it, believe it, and you can and will achieve it.

TRUE FITNESS STARTS FROM THE INSIDE OUT

This chapter takes a look at how my faith drives my fitness and the same can happen for you no matter what faith background you come from. This chapter is not here to preach, but for you to have an open mind to how the inner and outer fitness is tied together. You can read it or pass it over, but I sure hope you will have a look and receive some possible spiritual growth from it.

Owning your body works best from the inside out. You may be someone that internalizes your stress or many problems you might have in your life, even anger issues, job issues, family issues, and so on.

The people that take the time to come to terms with their inner peace and take time to pray often have a much better chance at achieving lasting fitness goals.

Stress takes your energy away from accomplishing productive things in your life, like your diet and fitness routine, or that business you wanted to start, or that class you wanted to take. Fitness from the inside out truly involves surrendering those worries to God, who can better handle the situation.

Fr. Nick Tocco is a priest in the Orlando Diocese and a enthusiastic gifted speaker, who enjoys working out. He once said in a public sermon to the congregation the following:

> "Faith is like being on a bench press and you're working to get that last final rep up and you're halfway there but you're stuck and you're sweating it out and the bar just isn't going anywhere, and then a guy will run over and give you a spot and help you make that final rep. Well, that's what it's like when you have faith in Christ. He will lift the bar and help you make the final rep."

Allowing your body to truly be fit from the inside out means you must get rid of all the anger, prejudices, hatred, disagreements, and gossips that you're holding on to and learn to forgive and accept differences and find solutions for the exercise of peace. There are ten good things that happen for every one bad thing and we must focus on the good. Don't let yourself be distracted by negative energy. Let prayer and internal fitness guide you to your outer fitness goals.

GOD'S PLAN: The Exercise of Faith

God gives His plans, which are many, to those that have a pure heart and a true love for Him. Having faith and counting on the Lord to help you in all areas of your life will help you to achieve your goals.

He often whispers to the common folk not to worry about all their imperfections. I remember when Christ appeared to me in a dream and when I opened my eyes, to my amazement, He was still there in the middle of the night on a 4th of July weekend, while I was visiting friends in Tampa, Florida. Every time I tell this story, I know people question it, but I must keep telling it because it is the truth and I have an obligation to tell it.

He was glowing white, like an angel but without wings, and the most beautiful sight I've ever laid eyes on. He said, "David, I love you," and when He pronounced my name, it sounded so very beautiful, in a way I'd never heard it sound before. Years later when I understood this vision more, I am sure it was a call to ministry that at the time I did not realize, but what I did know and believe is that His message was that of LOVE. It's that simple and has ALWAYS been that simple, although often communicated by so many as being so much more complicated. When I opened my eyes and He was still there, I felt my eyes to make sure they were open and they were. I was a bit overwhelmed and reached for the light switch. I turned the light on for a second, and then back off. Then the vision was gone, but the peace stayed and was on me. I used to think some of the religious shows on television with people falling down with the Holy Spirit on them and seeing them shaking was possibly not true, until I experience the electricity of the Holy Spirit on my own body and it is like an electricity tingling and pulling the skin, it is the most awesome feeling in the world and when your very much in tune with the Lord and open to what he has for you, this for sure can happen to you.

I remember this awesome presence of peace coming over my body. This is how you know for sure it's been a real experience. After laying there the rest of the night, I left very early the next morning and made my hour long drive back home in silence, wanting to hold on to that incredible feeling that had come over me. After that moment, and to this day still, I continue to open myself up to the work He may have for me to do. I often get great ideas that I know come from Him and it is up to me to put them into action and He will take it from there.

I wondered why I would be the one blessed with this dream. I mean, there are so many religious leaders out there that have never had this type of experience and yet I have, with all my imperfections that anyone could point a finger at. Yet, I have for all my life loved the Lord, believed without doubt in Heaven, prayed on a daily basis, attended church faithfully every Sunday since I can remember, attended Christian school, and have always felt that special love for God. But really, it's more simple than all of that because I, like many, am certainly no angel. God often gives His plan not to the great kings and queens and well known leaders but the common people that have more of a chance of fitting in and touching the lives of others.

The Lord actually came into this world homeless, and walked the earth not dressed up in a fancy cape and gown, but a simple robe and sandals. Look who He chose for his twelve apostles, very common men, even some He knew would betray Him due to their weakness of being human, yet He still chose them. He reached out to the sick, the persecuted, even those considered sinful. So I understand why it is He often comes to the regular everyday and not-so-everyday people like you and me. He has done this always, throughout His life when He was on this earth, yet so many even within the Christian faith, from believers to leaders within the churches, still miss the simple message of LOVE. DO NOT JUDGE, LET GOD JUDGE. Never ever tell someone they cannot enter the gates of Heaven, for only God can decide this, only God knows their heart and soul, not a mere observer like you and me. Spend your time building people up, not tearing them down like they did to Christ Himself. Remember, it has been said that the first will be the last, and the last will be the first.

So it makes much sense to me that God sometimes chooses those who others may not consider worthy. I believe Reverend Billy Graham offered the best perspective when he put it like this:

If you were God and you looked down on the earth and you saw this very special ant that you had given life to, headed for danger and there is a cliff that he will fall off of if he continues to follow the same path, you want to save him but the problem is how to do it. If you try to pick the ant up, you would squash it. If you put your finger down in front of it to stop it, the ant would crawl right over it. If you shout down from Heaven, you are sure to startle it. So, the only way to save the ant is to become an ant and communicate and warn the ant about the danger ahead with hopes of saving its life.

This is what God did when He sent His only Son into this world, not as a glorious king as some would have expected, but as a common folk. I believe this is why God still, most often, chooses to use people like you and me to spread His message and do His work.

No matter who you are and who I am, God is a God of love and a God of all! Even the New Catholic Pope Frances has been talking about this. He asks who is he to judge any person, no matter who they are, that seeks a personal relationship with God?- How true, since only God sees and reads a person's heart and soul, only he knows the real truth. God needs no Bible interpretations, he is the real thing. So let God play God and we will bow as his children and keep faith and love alive in him.

God provides us with miracles every day, yet when we hear of a miracle or know of someone that says they experienced one, we often doubt it, or read something of disbelief into it. Yet when the TV news channel, talk radio show, or a newspaper article only wants to spread gossipy half-truths, "political spin," and so on, most people are quick to believe in this without question. It's time to get our priorities in order. God is waiting to give out another miracle today, and it could be yours. Don't be afraid to ask for your miracle! Part of owning your body is also about owning your faith and spirituality too.

I remember when my business partner and I stepped out to start our business with no money and a lot of faith and trusted God to see us through. We made Him our business partner. So many people said we would fail, like many small start-up businesses do in their first six months. But we kept faith, worked hard and God blessed us. Here we are twenty years later, the proud owners of a business that helps people have a better quality of life.

If I had to pick my favorite and most exciting holiday, it would be Easter Sunday. The joy and enthusiasm of Christians all over the world is a very special feeling. There is a definite "spiritual energy" in the air.

On Easter morning, there is a feeling in my heart that touches my soul with my belief in the Resurrection of the Lord. It is the most important day of the year, yet overlooked by so many. On the following page, I have included a copy of my pastor's Easter message for all of you to read. I think there has never been a better definition of Easter than that which has been written by Monsignor Patrick J. Caverly, a truly gifted man. I hope this will touch you as it has touched me and possibly even bring a better understanding to those of you who may not have taken Easter Sunday as seriously as you should have. Read this message over twice and then share it with a friend.

My Dear Friends,

There is no day to compare with Easter Day. It stands out from the conflicts and turmoil of our broken world, lifts our minds, and enlivens our hearts with a joy and love so complete that it conquers death. Early on the first Easter morning, a mighty act of God took place — Christ rose from the dead, altered the past, and shaped the future. Nothing can be the same again. That is what makes Easter the greatest occasion of the year and Good News for all time. All our hopes and happiness stem from that event. Easter announces that there is a way forward out of darkness, transformation is possible, and change can take place in our lives.

The resurrection of Jesus from the dead affirms that death is not the end of us. We are meant for more than this present life and are not anchored to this world. Human life is no longer limited by the cycle of birth to death. Easter is the answer to all the tears that we shed at the graves of our loved ones because it reminds us that we have a future greater than we dare believe in, provided we open our hearts to the grace that Jesus won for us. Christ has shared the gift of His life with us, and His resurrection from the dead points to the resurrection of all people.

Easter is the turning point, inviting us to live in an entirely new way that goes beyond the limitations of this world. We are challenged to be part of a new creation, inspired by the life of God, which is poured into our souls at baptism. Life depends on how we look at it. It can be seen as an empty tomb, full of bitterness and confusion, or full of joy and hope. The challenge is to appreciate God and to see His plan in the ordinary events surrounding us. We can only do this if we are faithful to our baptismal promises, tuned into Jesus, and switched on to His power in our lives. He will help us to find the face of God in the bits and pieces of life and in the hearts of all whom we meet.

The Gospel tells us that on the first Easter morning, the stone at the entrance of the tomb of Christ was rolled back. The question we must all face is, Have we risen to a new life with Christ, or are there boulders weighing us down and keeping us imprisoned in our tombs? The best way we can give thanks to God for the gift of His life with us this Easter is by opening our hearts to the risen Jesus and by allowing ourselves to be sent out into the world to proclaim the good news of Christ's love.

May the joy of Easter be yours today and always!

Monsignor Patrick J. Caverly, V.G.
Church of the Annunciation

Do not allow differences in your relationships to cause

you to forget all the things you like about the relationship.

Different is good because it allows you

to exercise your mind and expand your views,

take in another's philosophies, and gain acceptance,

which leads to a fantastic fitness routine called

"Inner Growth"

CHAPTER EIGHT
OWNING THE ABILITY OF ACCEPTANCE

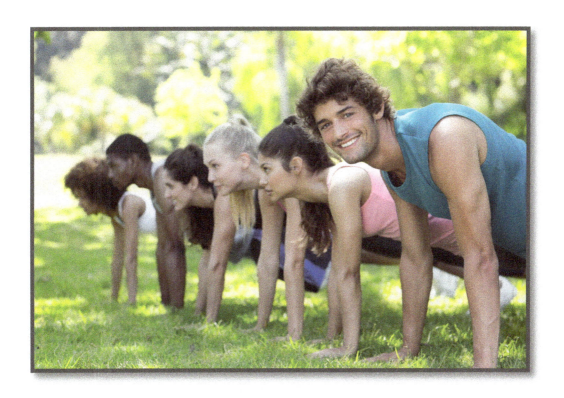

CHAPTER EIGHT
OWNING THE ABILITY OF ACCEPTANCE

If you are taking the time

to criticize others,

then this just means you

are not taking enough time

to improve yourself.

For if you give 100%

to being the best that you can be,

there will be no time to put others down.

This uses negative energy and creates

an atmosphere of failure, not success.

So be an example to others, be a leader, not a follower.

Shut down criticism, gossip, and bullying

when confronted with it.

Say something positive back

and this will extinguish the fire

that someone is trying to start.

Be that acceptance you seek.

GOD IS LOVE: Take ownership of God's love for you

GOD IS LOVE and He shows this love in many different forms and through many different people, which I call His "Angels on earth." This angel could be a doctor, friend, parent, teacher, pastor, policeman, fireman or a passing stranger.

GOD does not tear buildings down like what happened on 9/11. He builds them up. The devil tears buildings down by preying on the "self will" of humanity. When Christ spoke of how He could and would rebuild the temple in three days, He was not only speaking in a physical sense, but also of his spirit. We must focus on this and realize that buildings can fall, and our bodies can fall, but our spirit will live on and endure all circumstances because our soul belongs to GOD and even though the devil often attacks our physical beings, trying to shake our faith, nothing he does can affect our spiritual beings as long as we keep our faith in the Heavenly Father above.

In GOD's eyes, remember there is no death. That's how He can allow bad things to happen to good people's physical bodies. Because there is no death, the soul lives on in the glory of God forever and ever, as is the case with all who believe in Him.

It's all about FAITH, and where there is FAITH there is no room for fear. Fear has no value when you trust in the Lord Jesus Christ as your Savior, and His guarantee to each one of us, that believing in Him will give eternal and everlasting life.

One day we will leave this earth, some of us sooner than others. Make sure you live your years to the fullest and not necessarily the longest. There is a GOD and a devil, a Heaven and a hell, good and evil, and the choice is yours. Either you believe in GOD and His Son that died for our sins so that you may have everlasting life, or you believe in the other. But the truth is that Christ died for ALL people. The true message of Christianity is Heaven and not hell, and getting to Heaven needs to be our focus. Christ came not to condemn us, but to save us.

The choice is "cut and dry," so make the right choice today. We are all sinners and are saved by the blood of Christ. So remember, GOD loves you and He wants you in Heaven and He's saving a place for you and your loved ones. Exercise your FAITH today.

We all have an inner "invisible shield" given to us by GOD to protect us from harm and that shield is our soul. As long as we stay faithful to our Father in Heaven, then there is no need to worry because our soul is "indestructible." Our bodies may be physically able to be harmed, but our soul cannot be touched, and this is why through self-will that GOD allowed us to have as a people. He knows that sometimes devastation, sickness, and death may come to the physical body, but GOD puts His emphasis on the spiritual body, which is the part of us that will reign with Him for all of Eternity. There are many translations and interpretations of specific parts of the Bible. Some still stand today and others were a sign of the times and not parts of GOD's true love or it would have been part of the Ten Commandments or spoken of in detail by Christ. So we must not get so caught up in some of controversial parts that we miss the main message of GOD, the Father, Son, and Holy Spirit. It is about LOVE.

> The man who removes a mountain begins by carrying away small stones.

The following letter is from Monsignor Caverly on the subject of judgment. It appeared in one of our Sunday church bulletins and I felt it to be worthy of re-print in this book.

My Dear Friends,

All three readings today are concerned with our difficulty in understanding God's ways which always transcend what we are able to project or imagine. If the passage from Isaiah seems comfortably familiar and acceptable to us, that is because we have no difficulty with the proclamation that the Gentiles shall come into the inheritance of the Jews. We only have difficulties when we follow the principle further and realize that many are called to the Kingdom who are not members of our churches, who are not devout, who are not respectable. It is hard to take quite seriously the proposition that many who are now last in our own society and in our own esteem will be first, and that many who now are first in reputation and achievement will not fare so well.

How many are to be saved is not really our business to know in advance but we must know that it is a struggle like going through a very narrow door. Familiarity with tradition and worship is no guarantee of admission to the Kingdom. Some will come from far away and will be more readily welcomed. Salvation is by charity not by glib recitation of formulae nor even by assiduous performance of religious duties. Again and again, we find to our amazement, and perhaps to our chagrin, that the more disreputable and irreligious among us are those who are moved more profoundly by charity. Moreover, such movements of charity are often so spontaneous that it does not occur to such non-religious people to credit themselves with any virtue on account of compassionate and hospitable actions. This realization does indeed suggest a reversal of first and last.

To say that the first and the last will be reversed is to caution everyone about being too secure in their present position and to remind them that there is someone else who makes the final judgment. This parable is a warning to those in first place not to be presumptuous and to those in last place not to despair.

May God love you always!

Monsignor Patrick J. Caverly, V.G.
Church of the Annunciation

INVISIBLE CHAINS

There are so many still in today's society that are prejudiced in so many ways, in all segments of the population. They may be as big as a politician or preacher, or as common as the little town convenience worker or bus driver. But the world is getting more accepting as this new generation of 18 to 35 year olds have broken some of the chains of discrimination and are a much more open minded generation.

Not so long ago in history, the days of segregation echo in our recent past, when people of color had to sit at the back of the bus and could not share the same water fountains and restrooms with white folks and not even be allowed to sit in the same restaurants in some parts of the country. And to think that some of these people that allowed this segregation to occur actually thought of themselves as "Christians."

I hope we have come further than this today. But so many still put these "CHAINS" on different segments of the population and in so many ways we still have slavery even if it has taken on a different form or look. I call on everyone reading this book to perform a great exercise of removing these "Invisible Chains" from your way of life. We may not always agree with one another on all points of view, whether it is racial, gender, politics, religion, disabilities, lifestyle, etc. Times change and have we not learned that God made us all the same inside?

It's only the outer layer of skin that divides us. All of our blood is red, our internal organs are the same, our souls have no color, and pain and hurt have no color or gender. We must all accept God's unique plan for our own individuality. We can all point fingers and put each other down and pre-judge one another's lives. How simple and easy that would be, but the real question is can we all build each other up, love each other, encourage one another, pray for each other? Can we all be more like GOD who thought of all of these different segments of the population? To put each other down for any differences is to actually make fun of and be critical of God Himself for His blueprint of this world he created with all its differences. He could have made all the animals on this earth the same, all the fish in the sea the same, but he didn't because they all have a purpose on this earth.

If we were all perfect, we'd all be GOD, which would mean He could be replaced, which isn't his plan because no one can ever replace GOD. He wanted us to be more

Like Him, <u>NOT</u> HIM and he wanted the likeness to be in the form of LOVE.

Good things happen because God gives someone a plan and they put it into action. If we were all the same and had no differences then there would BE NO TEAM. Everyone's differences are a part of GOD'S TEAM. Almost like a football team, some are good at passing, others at receiving, some are good at kicking others at blocking and some have their strengths in coaching and so on.

If everyone were the same, with the same strengths in the same areas, then there would be no team, maybe all coaches and no players. The point is to accept each other's differences as strengths, NOT weaknesses, Strengths in GOD'S MASTER PLAN. He made each one of us, knows each one of us and loves each one of us with unconditional love. Lack of understanding one another's differences is in a way what CHRIST experienced when He was misunderstood and not accepted by many as the True Savior, and even then, He still reached his hand out to all the people.

GOD KNOWS US, HE KNOWS OUR "INDIVIDUALITY", EVEN WHEN OTHERS DON'T, AND HOW IT CAN BE THE BEST EXERCISE TO SUCCESS IN EACH OF OUR LIVES AND TO THE SUCCESS IN TEAM PLAY WHERE WE ALL WORK TOGETHER ON OUR INDIVIDUAL STRENGTHS, NOT OUR WEAKNESSES TO ACCOMPLISH A COMMON GOAL AND HOPEFULLY ONE DAY THAT GOAL WILL BE <u>PEACE ON EARTH</u> AND THE ACCEPTANCE OF EACH OTHER'S DIFFERENCES WITH UNCONDITIONAL LOVE FOR ONE ANOTHER. OWN YOUR INDIVIDUALITY TODAY AND ACCEPT THAT OF YOUR NEIGHBORS.

TAKE OWNERSHIP OF YOUR PET'S LOVE FOR YOU

We could all learn something from
our pets. If we all could treat each other
with the respect our dogs and cats use for us,
it would be a better world. Think about it …
Your pet doesn't worry about the color
of your skin, how much money you have,
your gender, what religion you embrace,
what political party you belong to,
how you dress, what type of car you drive,
the house you live in, how crabby you
are when you get home from work and so on …
And they always seem to forgive so fast
and they never talk bad about you!
Hmmm … Sounds like they're reaching out
in the teachings of the Lord
more so than a lot of humans.
I guess that is why dog is God spelled backwards.

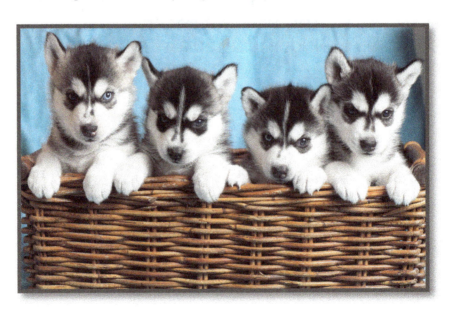

TAKE OWNERSHIP OF YOUR SELF CONTROL

Studies have shown that
One minute of anger produces
six hours of suppressed immunity.
Being angry can make you sick.

One minute of laughter produces
twenty-four hours of improved immunity.
Laughing actually makes you healthy.

Be slow to anger and
remember to have some fun.
Laugh and smile.
Take ownership of your self control.

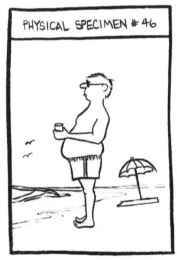

Charlie on the beach alone.

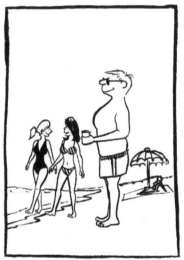

Charlie on the beach
with women around.

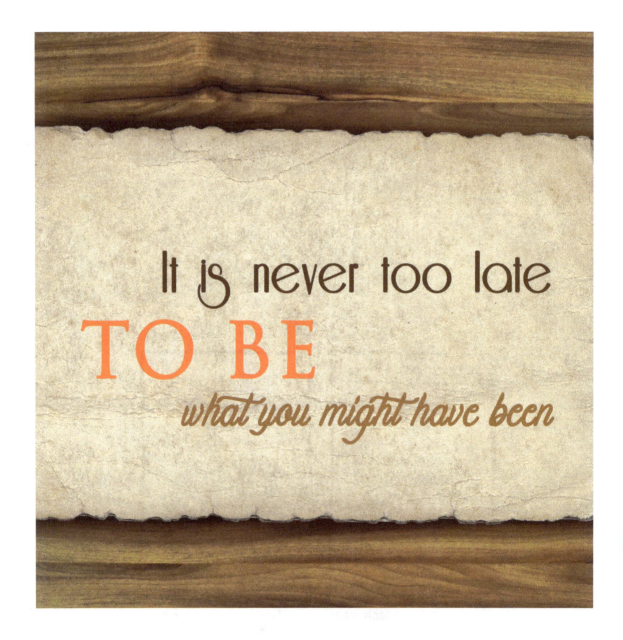

CHAPTER NINE
VITAMINS, HERBS, AND
ALTERNATIVE HEALTH PRODUCTS

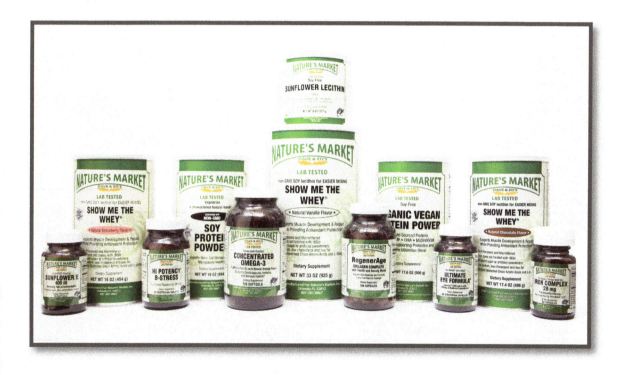

VITAMINS, HERBS, AND ALTERNATIVE HEALTH PRODUCTS

VITAMINS

	Functions
Vitamin A / Beta Carotene	* Maintenance of healthy skin, eyes, bones, hair and teeth * Beta Carotene is an antioxidant and can be converted by the body to vitamin A as needed
Vitamin D	* Assists in the absorption and metabolism of calcium and phosphorus for strong bones and teeth
Vitamin E	* As an antioxidant, helps protect cell membranes, lipoproteins, fats and vitamin A from destructive oxidation * Helps protect red blood cells * Take D-Alpha and not DL-Alpha which is synthetic
Vitamin K	* Needed for proper blood clotting
Vitamin C	* As an antioxidant, inhibits the formation of nitrosamines (a suspected carcinogen) * Important for maintenance of bones, teeth, collagen and blood vessels (capillaries) * Enhances iron absorption red blood cell formation * Best if taken in combination with Bioflavanoids
Vitamin B-1 (Thiamine)	* Releases energy from foods * Needed for normal appetite and for functioning of nervous system
Vitamin B-2 (Riboflavin)	* Releases energy from foods * Necessary for healthy skin and eyes

Vitamin B-3 (Niacin)	* Releases energy from foods
	* Aids in maintenance of skin, nervous system and proper mental functioning; can help with cholesterol
Vitamin B-6	* Releases energy from foods
	* Plays a role in protein and fat metabolism
	* Natural diuretic
	* Essential for function of red blood cells and hemoglobin synthesis
	* May help with carpel tunnel syndrome
Vitamin B-12	* Prevents pernicious anemia
	* Necessary for healthy nervous system
	* Involved in synthesis of genetic material (DNA)
Biotin	* Releases energy from foods
	* Plays a role in metabolism of amino acids
	* Needed for normal hair production and growth
Pantothenic Acid	* Releases energy from foods
	* Involved in synthesis of acetylcholine, an excitatory neurotransmitter
	* Needed for normal functioning of the adrenal glands
Folic Acid	* Necessary for proper red blood cell formation
	* Plays a role in the metabolism of fats, amino acids, DNA and RNA
	* Important for cardiovascular system and pre-natal
	* Needed for proper cell division and protein synthesis
Choline	* As a liptropic nutrient, prevents fat accumulation in the liver
	* Precursor to acetylcholine, a major neurotransmitter in the brain
Inositol	* Involved in calcium mobilization

MINERALS

	Functions
Boron	* Possibly plays a role in maintaining strong bones * Affects calcium and magnesium metabolism * May be needed for proper membrane function
Calcium	* Builds strong bones and teeth * Involved in nerve transmission and muscle contraction * Use Calcium Citrate for better absorption
Chromium	* As part of Glucose Tolerance Factor (GTF), it works with insulin to regulate blood sugar levels
Copper	* Essential for red blood cell formation, hemoglobin synthesis * Involved in many enzyme systems, including super oxide dismutase (SOD), a major antioxidant enzyme system
Iodine	* Needed for proper functioning of the thyroid gland and production of thyroid hormones
Iron	* Prevents anemia; as a constituent of hemoglobin, transports oxygen throughout the body
Magnesium	* Needed in many enzyme systems, especially those involved with energy production * Essential for proper heartbeat and nerve transmission * Constituent of bones and teeth
Manganese	* Cofactor in many enzyme systems including those involved in bone formation, energy production, and protein metabolism
Molybdenum	* Required for proper growth and development * Plays a role in fat and nucleic acid metabolism * Needed for proper sulfur metabolism
Phosphorus	* Maintains strong bones and teeth * Necessary for muscle and nerve function

Potassium	* An electrolyte needed to maintain fluid balance, proper heartbeat and nerve transmission
Selenium	* As an antioxidant, it is a constituent of glutathione peroxidase * Protects vitamin E
Silicon	* Needed for proper bone structure and growth
Zinc	* Component of insulin required for blood sugar control * Needed for proper taste and hearing * Important in wound healing and enzyme activation * Important for men's reproductive system.

Healthy Hint: B vitamins work best when all are taken together. Very important for those in stress situations. Vital to your entire glandular system, especially the adrenal glands. So it is highly recommended that you take a B-complex rather than just individual B vitamins.

Healthy Hint: Lecithin granules are important to your health. All the cells and organs have lecithin surrounding them for protection. Take a serving with your first meal of the day or add it to a smoothie. Lecithin is also heart healthy for cholesterol and liver cleansing.

Healthy Hint: Zinc is very important for immune system support, but only up to 100mg daily with the average dose being 30mg-50mg. Anything over 100 mg actually depletes the immune system and is doing the complete opposite of what you are trying to do.

Vitamin C

So simple, yet so powerful. Vitamin C is an antioxidant and is required for approximately 300 functions of the body. This includes tissue growth and repair, gland function, healthy gums along with aiding in anti-stress, immune system response and the metabolism of other vital vitamins and amino acids.

Taking Vitamin C has been shown in studies to reduce symptoms of asthma, protect against pollution, prevent cancer, guard against infection, reduce and help eliminate toxic substances from the body, lower bad cholesterol, lower blood pressure, form collagen in the skin, protect against blood clotting and bruising, heal wounds and burns, fight free radicals in the bloodstream and much more.

The body cannot manufacture Vitamin C. So it must be gotten through your diet. Vitamin C works well with Vitamin E and Beta-Carotene and should be taken combined with bio-flavonoids to help with absorption. I highly recommend Vitamin C for everyone to take, especially those with chronic illnesses. Take in divided dosages and in buffered form to protect stomach lining. Vitamin C should be taken separate from aspirin; pregnant women should not exceed 5,000 mg. per day. The Calcium Ascorbate form or Ester-C form are the best.

Vitamin E

Vitamin E is an antioxidant that plays an important role in the prevention of cardio-vascular disease and cancer. It is known for improving circulation, tissue repair and is good for premenstrual syndrome and fibrocystic disease affecting breast.

Vitamin E promotes normal blood clotting and healing, helps reduce scarring, reduces blood pressure, helps in the prevention of cataracts and relaxes leg cramps. It is very important for healthy nerves and is needed for healthy skin and hair. Studies show it may slow the progression of Alzheimer's disease and may protect against over eighty different diseases.

Vitamin E prevents cell damage and the formation of free radicals. It helps fight against age spots and in some cases even in the prevention of heart attacks.

Vitamin E is best in it's natural form rather than synthetic. Natural is listed as D-alpha and synthetic is listed as dl-alpha, which makes it much less active than natural Vitamin E.

If you are on blood thinners do not take more than 400 I.U's of Vitamin E daily. If you have diabetes, heart disease, high blood pressure or thyroid conditions do not take over the recommenced amount and check with your physician.

Miatake Mushroom

This mushroom has been labeled the "king of all mushrooms" and grows wild in Japan and parts of North America.

It's been a part of Chinese and Japanese herbology for many years and is known for helping strengthen the immune system due to its incredible healing properties.

There is a very special polysaccharide contained in the Miatake called Beta-1, 6-Glucan, which is very powerful. In fact in some laboratory studies this substance has been shown to inhibit the growth of cancerous tumors, kill HIV cells and enhance key immune cells known as the T-helper cells or CD4 cells. Miatake is better utilized when taken with Vitamin C and dosages may vary depending on illness or if it's just being taken as an everyday immune boosting supplement.

IP-6 (Inositol Hexaphosphate)

This powerful antioxidant has many positive effects on the body and is a compound consisting of the B Vitamin Inositol plus six phosphate groups. I find laboratory studies very exciting on IP-6 because it has been shown that it may fight cancer and even may block the spread of the cancer from the bad cells to the good cells when taken in high dosages. Some other studies also suggest it to be beneficial in heart disease, liver disease and kidney stones.

IP-6 works so well because it seems to inhibit the activity of free radicals, which, in turn, slows abnormal cell division associated with cancer and tumor growth. IP-6 contains Beta-1,3-D-Glucan, which helps to promote a strong immune system especially in people undergoing chemotherapy and radiation. There's even an additional benefit to IP-6 and that is it protects the heart by possibly preventing blood clots to form in the blood vessels and by reducing levels of cholesterol and triglycerides in the bloodstream. Studies have shown that IP-6 may reduce the risk of cancer especially in the breast, colon and prostate.

Noni Juice

This very special fruit grown in Tahiti and also known by the name Morinda Citrifolia, has been known for being an incredible immune booster with only one to two ounces needed per day to see some outstanding health benefits. The following are some of the testimonies I've heard about and gladly pass on to you.

Today, people are using 100% Pure Noni for a broad spectrum of ailments including:

* High blood pressure	* Headaches	* Diabetes
* Menstrual cramps	* Hypoglycemia	* Diarrhea
* Arthritis	* Other inflammatory diseases	* Fever
* Constipation	* Other gastrointestinal problems	* Coughs
* Circulation	* Mouth and throat infections	* Jaundice
* Depression		

Shark Cartilage

This substance is classified as a food supplement and is actually made from the skeleton of sharks.

I find this product to be very interesting and in some individuals it has been very helpful when taken in proper dosage and quality.

The very important part of shark cartilage is that it actually works to suppress the development of new blood vessels. You may ask why this is so very important and it is because many cancerous tumors only grow because they live off of blood as their main nutrient, and if the tumor can be cut off from the blood source, well there's a good chance it will shrink up.

Another part of shark cartilage that I find to be beneficial is to those suffering from Diabetic Retinopathy and Macular Degeneration, that are supported by the growth of new blood vessels which can lead to blindness. I saw this in my mother when she was suffering from Macular Degenerations and she had blood vessels bursting behind her eyes, the doctor wanted to do laser surgery to get this to stop. I however put her on the shark cartilage and it did stop the blood vessel formation. She ended up not needing that particular surgery.

Other uses for shark cartilage are in the treatment of Arthritis, Psoriasis and Bursitis (that would be in the shoulder typically).

I recommend only Benefin Shark Cartilage from Lane Labs – this is a very pure source.

Shark Cartilage should not be used by persons who have recently undergone surgery or have had a heart attack. It also should not be used by pregnant women and children.

Coenzyme Q 10

This vitamin-like substance is considered a powerful antioxidant and has certain properties that resemble that of Vitamin E. Coenzyme Q 10 is the only one of the Coenzyme Q's family that is actually found in human tissue and plays an important part in the production of energy to every cell in our bodies, which in turn increases tissue oxygenation to stimulate our immune system, aid in circulation and even stimulate anti-aging effects.

CO-ENZYME Q 10 has been noted for its treatment and prevention of cardiovascular disease. Scientists conducted studies and have shown up to a 75% chance of survival in congestive heart failure cases when Co-Enzyme Q 10 was added to their conventional therapy treatments. Since Co-Enzyme Q 10 strengthens the heart muscle, it has been widely used in Japan by more than 12 million people upon direction by their physicians. Other diseases that show benefits from this substance are Alzheimer's disease, cardiovascular disease, multiple sclerosis, periodontal disease, diabetes and muscular dystrophy. 50-150 mg. in soft gel form is recommended per day. After age 30, CO-Q10 levels start to decline, and with insufficient CO-Q10 the cells don't make energy to sustain life. CO-Q10 is used by all cells in the body. UBIQUINOL is considered a superior choice.

MSM (Methylsulfonylmethane)

This is a naturally occurring organic sulfur compound found in plant and animal tissues that is very important for overall health. I have found in my work that it has really helped a lot of my customers that suffer from muscle pain, arthritis, immune problems and even heartburn. MSM also helps hair, skin and nails but is best known for relieving pain and inflammation. You can usually see benefits from MSM in anywhere from three to twenty-five days and in a dosage that starts out with 1,000 mg. the first week and increases anywhere from 2,000-3,000 mg. per day in divided dosages with food. I suggest taking it with Vitamin C to aid in absorption.

Alpha-Lipoic Acid

I find this antioxidant both powerful and exciting because of its tremendous health benefits that I have seen first-hand in how it has helped several of my customers. There are two major benefits in taking Alpha-Lipoic Acid, the first is that it helps balance and lower sugar levels in diabetics because it is known as a Metabolic Antioxidant. Without it cells cannot use sugar to produce energy. Alpha-Lipoic Acid is considered one of the best overall antioxidants. It is also said to help the liver.

Glucosamine-Sulfate and Chondroitin Sulfate

Glucosamine and Chondroitin have really helped a lot of people that suffer from arthritis. In fact I've actually seen some of my customers not end up needing knee replacement surgeries after one year on this wonderful natural substance.

Glucosamine has been proven in over 300 studies to actually build joint cartilage and to reduce the destruction of cartilage, along with having anti-inflammatory properties. Chondroitin sulfate tends to provide a cushion in the joints and even though a much larger molecule than Glucosamine Sulfate, the two together seem to have had amazing effects on many people suffering from arthritis and osteoarthritis.

It is recommended that approximately 1500 mg. of Glucosamine Sulfate be consumed per day and some benefits will be seen within one month's time. However the longer you stay on the product the better. I recommend consuming this product for at least one to two years for best results since it rejuvenates approximately 30% of your cartilage per year, which is a lot when you consider all the years it took you to break down the cartilage. This product is considered safe for the most part. But you may want to check with your physician if you are taking any medications, especially blood thinners since Chondroitin can thin the blood and you may use Glucosamine by itself. I recommend ARTH-MAX Liquid by Olympia Health, with which my customers have had great results, or the Lifetime Liquid Glucosamine Formula.

Calcium Citrate

This form of calcium has proven to have a much higher absorption rate than that of calcium carbonate. In fact anyone over the age of fourty should take calcium in the citrate form because as we age, we produce less and less digestive enzymes to break down a carbonate form of calcium. Take only quality tested brands from your health food stores in the range of 1,000-1,500 mg. of calcium with approximately 500 mg. of magnesium and some Vitamin D taken in divided dosages. If you wish to take one mega dose before bed it will help you sleep. However, your absorption would be better divided up.

Remember that menopausal women, female athletes, and pregnant women all need calcium supplements. Research has indicated a link in the ageing process that ties lowering of estrogen levels as women age to loss of bone density. I personally believe that men also lose bone density as they age due to lower testosterone levels. But their loss of bone density doesn't seem to be as severe as the women. However, some level of calcium supplementations would prove to also be beneficial to them.

Calcium deficiency has been linked to bone and teeth problems, aching joints, nail problems, eczema, high cholesterol, hypertension, muscle cramps and osteoporosis.

It is suggested to take calcium that also has magnesium with it. Some studies have shown that calcium tends to absorb magnesium out of the body and this may lead to an actual magnesium deficiency if it is not taken with the calcium. Bluebonnet Liquid Calcium Citrate with Magnesium is an excellent choice.

Colostrum

I have found this product to be quite interesting and have received several testimonials from customers on how it has improved several health conditions.

What is Colostrum? Well it's found to be a "non-milk" material found in breast milk. It's actually secreted by the mammary glands of all female mammals in the last months of pregnancy. Now this is why breast-feeding seems to be a very important part of the immune system during the first few days after being born. Colostrum is, for most newborns, their very first meal that contributes to building their entire immune system. Calf's Colostrum closely resembles human Colostrum and offers similar benefits.

Here are some cases that Colostrum has been considered effective in helping;

Rheumatoid arthritis, MS, Lupus, Type I Diabetes, Graves Disease, allergies, exposure to toxins, Auto-Immune Diseases, infections, chronic Fatigue Syndrome, and overall immune enhancement. Colostrum has also been shown to release IGF-1 growth factors, which contribute to the function of growth hormone in the body. New growth hormone has been shown to have anti-aging properties, increase muscularity and speed-up metabolism for fat loss. Colostrum is also believed to speed-up the repair and recovery of the body and muscle groups. There haves been testimonies from individuals suffering from cancer, heart disease, eczema, obesity, eye problems, colon and intestinal problems, T-Cell suppression and many other health concerns. I recommend Immune Tree Colostrum 6 as a quality brand to consume. For more information on colostrum pick up a copy of "Colostrum" by Lance S. Wright, M.D.

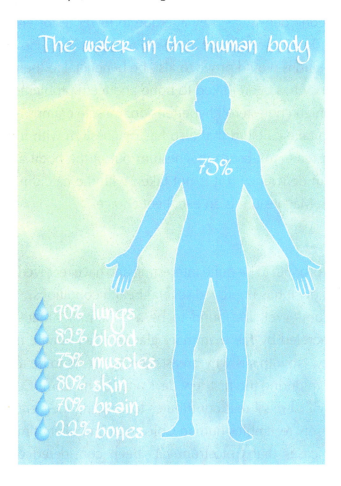

Colon Cleansing

Colon cleansing could be the one most important thing you can do to protect your health.

Most people will go their entire lives without ever cleansing their colon. This part of the human body in many cases holds the key to our overall health. However, it tends to be ignored by most.

Several studies show that many diseases start within the wall of the colon and work their way up into other organs as far-reaching as even the brain.

The most toxic colon and intestinal walls are found in those persons that consume diets high in red meat and pork. And also low in fiber and low in water consumption.

Cleansing the colon at least twice per year is very important. The best time to remember to do a cleanse is in April and October when the time changes. Most cleanses take about two weeks to complete and are very simple to follow. The first couple days you may experience some gentle detoxifying effects, but then you will start to feel refreshed and re-energized.

I recommend the Nature's Secret Ultimate Cleanse product, which is simple to use, you take two pills upon rising and two pills before bed with a full glass of water. This product will help cleanse your heart, kidneys, lungs, blood and colon along with allowing for approximately five pounds or more of easy weight loss just from getting the build-up of "Gook" off your intestinal wall and colon.

Picture never brushing your teeth, EVER, your whole life, meal after meal. Imagine the build-up of plaque and food particles that you would have. Pretty disgusting thought, isn't it?

Well, multiply that thought several times over again and you'll get the picture of what your intestine and colon will look like if it's never been cleansed.

Remember cleansing your intestinal wall and colon could actually be the difference between life and death. It's one of the best things you can do for yourself and the best health advice you can pass on to your loved ones.

You'll be able to feel the difference and you'll be glad you took this major step in preserving your health.

Black Seed Oil - This is a potent immune system booster and was said to even be found in the tomb of King Tut, It is said that it showed that even with all the gold and things of kings he could have taken to his tomb, he chose black seed oil to be taken with him into his next life, showing the value it held with him in that day and age as a priceless possession. Black seed oil contains over 100 natural chemical compounds and was even featured on the Dr. Oz show for its' impressive immune system boosting properties which include: anti-cancer, anti-bacteria, anti-histamine, anti-inflammatory, anti-parasitic,

Anti-Acne and more, with just one teaspoon full per day mixed with one teaspoon of raw honey or juice and taken on an empty stomach 30-60 minutes before food. In more serious cases it can be used up to three times per day under a health care professional's guidance and never exceed three servings per day.

Moringa - Nicknamed by some the finger of God and by others the miracle tree. It seems to have endless health benefits and anti-aging properties. Many uses are being studied for this wonderful tree remedy, but so far it seems to have very impressive properties that include: Anti-Tumor, Anti—Diabetic, Anti-Microbial, Anti-Inflammatory, Anti-Viral and a strength to increase immunity against several different diseases. The Natural News has called it the "Ultimate Super-food" on their web site: www.naturalnews.com.

.

ASTRAGALAS	Popular for its overall immune boosting properties. Helps to fight bacteria, parasites, and fungus. Helps shorten the duration of a cold.
BILBERRY	Has been shown to improve eye function, including night vision, macular degeneration, glaucoma, cataracts, and diabetes.
BLACK COHOSH	Has been used to improve hot flashes, menopausal symptoms, and menstrual cramps.
BURDOCK ROOT	This herb has been used in the treatment of blood cleansing, acne, cancer, gout, fluid retention, and hemorrhoids.
CASCARA SAGRADA	Mostly used for constipation as a laxative. This herb should be used with caution if you have any health problems such as irritable bowel syndrome or colitis.
CAYENNE PEPPER	Used for poor circulation and topically in cream form for arthritis pain.
CRANBERRY	Excellent for bladder infections, kidney stones, and is a urinary acidifier.
DANDELION	Mostly used for fluid retention and swelling, also good for gout, kidney stones, and heavy metal toxins.
DONG QUAI	Very useful for menstrual cramps, hot flashes, and overall female tonic.

ECHINACEA	This very popular herb is great for cold season, works well as an antibacterial, anti viral, immune booster. This herb is best taken no more than 2-3 weeks at a time and then give yourself a one-week break. Good for colds, coughs, lymph node swelling, sinus, sore throat, ear infections, and more. Check with your physician before taking if you have any autoimmune disease such as tuberculosis, HIV, or multiple sclerosis, since in these cases it may be shown to aggravate certain conditions. Overall Echinacea has been shown to be safe for adults, children and even pregnant women.
FEVERFEW	Excellent for headaches, fever, migraines, and muscle strain.

Heathy Tip: Elderberry(Sambucus) is effective against flu viruses, lowers fever and relieves cough and congestion. This immune enhancer is something you should keep in your cabinet especially if anyone else around you is sick, it can also work as a preventive.

GARLIC	This herb works well as an anti-bacterial, anti-fungal, anti-yeast, and natural immune boosting anti-biotic. This should be consumed as a part of your everyday diet. Make sure that the garlic you purchase is cold processed, odor controlled, and has a high Allicin content. Excellent for colds, flu, yeast, blood pressure, cholesterol, auto immune problems, sinusitis, diabetics, parasite infection, fungal infections, thrush, and much more.
GINGER	Used for upset stomach, motion sickness, colds, low blood sugar, laryngitis and much more.

GINKO BILOBA	This herb is popular for memory, it's known for increasing the blood flow through the brain, which allows you to remember better. This herb has been good for helping with Alzheimer's disease, asthma, stroke, circulation, and other ailments. This herb can thin the blood so check with your physician if you're taking any anti-clotting drugs.
GREEN TEA	This herb has been shown to improve the immune system and has excellent antioxidant properties, anti-cancer properties, and cardiovascular benefits as well. If taken in capsule form, try to get an extract that contains 80 percent polyphenol.
GYMNEMA SYLVESTRE	Known for its benefits of balancing sugar levels in the body, used by persons with both high and low sugar levels. This herb also reduces glucose in the urine and helps suppress the taste for sugar.
HAWTHORN	Great for strengthening the heart muscle and is also good for angina, high blood pressure, palpitations, heart failure and stroke.
HORSETAIL	Known for its natural Silica properties that help to improve the hair, skin and nails. This herb is best taken three months on and one month off since it can irritate the kidneys in sensitive individuals. This herb taken with biotin has given some very good results for thickening the hair.
KAVA KAVA	Used mostly for its calming effects on the nerves. Helps to promote relaxation. This herb should not be used with alcohol and check with your physician if you are on any anti-depressants. Three months on, one off to protect liver enzyme elevation.
KELP	Excellent for persons with under-active thyroids, obesity and also has a lot of minerals naturally occurring as do most sea plants.

Healthy Hint: Maca Root increases energy, helps with fatigue and improves intimacy in both men and woman.

MILK THISTLE	This herb has some great properties to it and is greatly known for its detoxifying effects on the liver. Generally regarded as safe, this herb is beneficial for persons having to detoxify from alcoholism, heavy metal toxins, radiation, heavy amounts of medications, steroids, and anyone working with toxic chemicals on a daily basis.
MULLIEN	Works well for asthma, colds, coughs, bronchitis, emphysema, and congestion in the chest.
PAUL D'ARCO	Anti-fungal, anti-tumor, anti-viral, anti-bacterial, and anti-flammatory. Works well for yeast and fungal infections.
RED CLOVER	Anti-cancer, digestant, estrogenic, hastens tissue renewal, good for acne, cancer, eczema, lymph node, swelling, psoriasis, stomach cancer, promotes bile flow. This herb may thin the blood, do not take with blood-thinner.
RED RASBERRY LEAF	Used successfully in many cases to shorten the labor time in mothers that are delivering babies. Also helps with menstrual bleeding and cramps.
ST. JOHNS WORT	A very popular herb for depression and stress. This herb also works as an anti-bacterial. It is best if taken at a dosage of 900 mgs. per day of extract and 0.3% hypericin. If you are sensitive to the sun then you need to be careful while on this herb since it can make you burn more easily. Check with your physician if you are on any anti-depressants.

SAW PALMETTO	This herb has been wonderful for those suffering from prostate enlargement in the benign state and also for overall health of the prostate. This herb also works in cases of bladder infection, hair thinning or loss and impotence.
SIBERIAN GINSENG	Used mostly as a stimulant for energy and circulation. Has been shown to help in Alzheimer's, fatigue, depression, impotence, memory, low blood sugar and other ailments. This herb can cause insomnia if taken too late and can also be too stimulating for those with high blood pressure.
STINGING NETTLE	This herb has worked for allergies, asthma, hay fever, coughs, hives, benign prostate symptoms, thinning hair, and has anti-inflammatory properties.
TEA TREE	Used in many natural products as an antiseptic and anti-fungal. This product should not be swallowed and is used mostly as an external application for cuts, scrapes, nail fungus, boils and is used as a mouth rinse for abscesses, canker sores and is found in several natural toothpastes at your local health food stores.
VALERIAN ROOT	This herb is used mostly at bedtime to help relaxation and to promote sleep. This herb should not be used in high dosages during waking hours and should be avoided when driving. It has also been used for stress, migraines, jet lag, and for attention deficit disorder in lower dosages and also for restless leg syndrome. This herb should not be taken more than three months without getting off of it for one month since it may cause kidney irritations in sensitive individuals.
WHITE WILLOW BARK	Known for its anti-inflammatory properties, this herb resembles aspirin and has been used for joint pain, arthritis, sore throat, teething, toothaches, and menstrual cramps.

MY TOP PICKS FOR GOOD HEALTH

Green Vibrance

This greens drink product is made by Vibrant Health. It is one of the best green supplements on the market. Green Vibrance contains 25 billion probiotics, organic greens, and freeze-dried grass juices. This product helps each cell in the body to work at its peak immunity and energy level. It will detox and restore, along with balancing pH levels in the body. It is a top super food. Perfect for daily use and also for those persons needing to jump-start their immune systems after illness or just as a preventative and good health maintenance product. I highly recommend you try it.

Vitamin D-3

Such a simple vitamin holds a power pack of health and has gotten a lot of attention in the last year or so. The health benefits of vitamin D-3 have now come out as being amazing. Vitamin D-3 is made from Cholecalciferol and when we are in the sun, however, not to the degree that is shown to have major medicinal properties. There is for sure health benefits to safe sun exposure, but to get the levels you would need for some major health changes, it would be recommended to take at least 1,000 IU of Vitamin D-3, which is what was used in the studies showing a possible help with decreasing cancer cells, depression, heart disease, dementia, and more. The average dose is 1,000 to 5,000 IU per day, some doctors are prescribing even more and they are now looking at these levels when your blood work is taken. This gained recent exposure on a popular doctor of health television show.

Flaxseed Oil

This wonderful health oil is rich in Omega 3, 6 & 9. It supplies approximately 6200 mg of Omega 3 per tablespoon which is equal to six fish oil pills. This rich oil is known for helping lower blood pressure, cholesterol, helping with memory, focus, hormone balance, skin problems, arthritis, inflammation, and also is a fat emulsifier. It is kind of like putting oil in your car, it makes the engine run, it lubricates from the inside out. I recommend this product.

Red Yeast Rice

Impressive results have been seen by many using this product for lowering cholesterol. It has a natural statin property. It also must be taken in a citrinin-free form and works best adding Co-Q10 since statins deplete this in the body. This product is best taken three months on and one month off and the suggested dose is 600mg taken twice daily. I have had some customers experience amazing results in lowering cholesterol, especially when adding it with the flaxseed oil or fish oil.

Blood Pressure Factors

Most likely one of the best products with which I have had experience in lowering my customers' blood pressure. This product is put out by Michael's and has a complete blend of natural products to lower blood pressure. It is taken three times a day and can be taken with your medication or trial used prior to going on the medication. Once the blood pressure is stable, you may be able to slowly come off the medication under a doctor's care and go totally on this wonderful natural product. We have sold it consistently for over twelve years and have seen it work, especially when taken with flaxseed oil.

Thymulus

By Enzymatic Therapy, a product that every household should have. It is one of my favorite daily immune boosters, especially if you work around a lot of people. This product supports our thymus gland, which is the center of our immune system. It contains raw thymus and astragalas root extract. It is a super immune booster.

Beta-Glucan

Wow, this Beta-1,3 glucan enhances the natural macrophage activity, which is an integral part of and the most competent cell known to our immune system. I have seen people restore their health using this product and it has been shown to possibly have anti-cancer activity and is capable of re-booting the immune system.

Mega Food Multi Vitamin

All good nutrition starts with a multi-vitamin. The secret to a good multi is it must be whole-food based for proper absorption and 100% is even better. The Mega Food line provides this for men, women, and children. It only contains what was naturally in the fruits and vegetables that were squeezed and put into tablet form. Your body will recognize this as a food, digest it like a food, and is one of the few multi-vitamins that is gentle enough to even be taken on an empty stomach. There are no harsh fillers or tough coatings that don't allow the vitamin to break down like you will find in grocery store brands. This vitamin has superior absorption. One of my favorites.

Fema Max

This is one of the best natural menopause formulas on the market today and includes a blend of herbs and a natural hormone that will balance hot flashes and estrogen levels. I have carried this product for many years and women constantly come back for it and give their personal testimony on how much it has helped them with just the first bottle's 30-days worth.

Prostate Formula

By Nature's Market. This is a specialty prostate formula that we have produced especially for our customers, using the best ingredients known for prostate health all in one formula. It is a complete blend that helps re-balance the prostate gland for overall health. I have had customers that thought they were going to need surgery, but after just one month on this formula there was major improvement. I strongly suggest it for anyone having prostate issues, frequent urination, swollen prostate, E.D., or high PSA test showing problems. This is a must-have for any men of forty or over. The prostate is the second leading cause of death in men after heart disease. Take it seriously.

Colloidiol Silver

I recommend Silver Biotics Brand. This Silver product is a natural antibiotic and really supports the wellness of the body, while treating so many health issues. The great thing about taking this natural antibiotic is that it only kills the bad bacteria in the body and allows the good bacteria to grow and still fight for your good health. This product I have carried for years and it is also something everyone should have in their homes.

Customers love it and it truly works when taken right and in the proper parts per million strength. Silver Biotics offers it in a 10ppm and it is also good in nasal spray for sinus infection in a product called Nasal Rescue by Peaceful Mountain. This product is great for colds, infections, sore throats, skin problems, and much more. It also comes in a topical gel. It is actually said to be on trial in some of the veterans' hospitals. It is important to get quality brands in your local health food store.

Oscillococcinum

Another of my favorites. This product is put out by Boiron and is simply the best flu product you can take if started within the first 48 hours of symptoms. It is a natural homeopathic remedy so it is safe, and is available in both adult and children's formulas. This product fights flu, chills, body aches, fatigue, headaches, all the above when it is flu related. You take one vial under the tongue every six hours. This should be in everyone's household and in every suitcase when traveling.

Pain Max Cream

This product is put out by Olympia Health and works wonders for arthritis pain, inflammation, muscle pulls and injuries. It is applied topically with a high absorption transport method right to the area hurting. It contains Arnica and a blend of natural ingredients. It has a pleasant almond smell, non-greasy, and can be used as needed. This gets right to the problem and does not just cover it up like the heat rub products do.

Goldenseal Extract

This is a popular herb introduced by Native Americans. Goldenseal is considered a natural antibiotic and can only be used for one week at a time. It is good for sore throats, especially at the first sign of getting one, also for colds, infections, sinus and chest congestion and has many other secondary uses as well. I recommend the extract capsule form from Solaray for getting the job done well.

DGL

Deglycyrrhizinated licorice. This chewable herbal supplement can be used to treat heartburn, acid reflux, indigestion, and also has been shown to benefit ulcerated stomach linings. DGL increases the protective mucus coating in the intestinal tract, the stomach, and esophagus. I recommend Enzymatic Therapy or Natural Factors brand. Chew two tablets before or between meals. Check with your physician if you are being treated for any serious health conditions. For the most part, it is usually tolerated very well and is not to be confused with licorice candy. It is not the same thing.

Acidophilus and Probiotic Supplements

Acidophilus is a friendly probiotic bacteria that is found in the intestinal tract. It supports the digestive system, immune system, and is very important for anyone taking or coming off of antibiotics. This product will restore the good bacteria that is killed from the antibiotics. Acidophilus also helps fight yeast infections, urinary tract infections, diarrhea, and many other ailments. It is available in the refrigerated section of health food stores and also comes in a shelf-stable version. Make sure the potency is guaranteed on the label.

What should you take for your basics

Woman:
Women's 100% whole food based multi one a day, Biosil from Natural Factors, Ester Vit C500, B-Complex 100, Evening Primrose Oil or Flax Oil, Damiana/Ginseng blend from Solaray, Whey Protein shake and a super greens powder such as Perfect Food-Raw.

Woman 40+ :
Woman's 100% whole food based multi one a day, Biosil, Ester C500, Evening Primrose or Flax Oil, B-Complex 100, Fema-Max with DHEA from Natural Max (or 7keto DHEA), Calcium Citrate, Whey Protein shake, and a supper greens powder such as Perfect Food-Raw. (DHEA is a hormone, take 7 Keto DHEA as a non hormone substitute, both available in health food stores for individuals in good health.)

Men:

Men's 100% whole food multi one a day, Ester C500, B-Complex 100, Zinc, Omega 3 Fish Oil or Flax Oil, Whey Protein Shake, super greens food such as Perfect Food- Raw and Tribulus 500mg.

Men 40+:

Men's 100% whole food multi one a day, Ester C500, B-Complex 100, Zinc, Omega 3 Fish Oil or Flax Oil, DHEA 25-50mg or 7keto DHEA, Whey Protein shake, super greens powder such as Perfect Food-Raw and Testo-Extreme from Olympia Health, or Male Response by Source Naturals.

Individuals with immune system problems:

Whole Food Based Multi-Vitamin

Ester C- 1,000 mg per day.

Vitamin D-3 1,000mg

Beta Glucan -200 mg per day

Flax Seed Oil- One tablespoon per day

Thymulus from Enzymatic Therapy- 2 pills per day

Super Green Foods Drink-Perfect Food, Once per day

Whey Hydrolyzed Protein Shake- gf/df one per day.

*As with any health issues, please consult your physician for advice on your individual needs since you health care advisor will be able to guide you best from your specific health history and lab work.

ANTIOXIDANTS AND FREE RADICALS

What are they? Well, antioxidants are natural compounds that protect the body from harmful free radicals. These are groups of atoms that cause damage to the cells, the immune system and can lead to various diseases, infections and cancer. There is also substantial evidence that free radical damage plays a role in the aging process.

Free radicals are known to occur in the body from several different sources including: exposure to toxic chemicals, cigarette smoke, pollution, industrial and household chemicals and various other sources. These free radicals are seen in the bloodstream under a microscope as black particles floating around in our blood breaking down our cellular walls, which in turn slowly break down our immune system. When we consume antioxidants such as Vitamins A, Beta Carotene, C, E and Selenium to name a few, this helps our cells to destroy the free radicals before they destroy the cells, it's like giving our cells the ammunition they need to win the battle.

Free radicals are for real, they are attacking our system every day. There are certain natural clinics that you can go to and they can do a prick blood test and put your blood under a scope and flash it up onto a screen and you will actually see the cells attacking the free radicals, you will be amazed just how much life there is in just a drop of blood and all the activity that is going on to make your body work.

Healthy Fact: Did you know that the body is made up of two-thirds water and that you should consume eight 8-ounce glasses of water just for proper body functioning of all your internal organs. Many people are dehydrated and do not know it.

Health Note: A poll of 37,000 Americans sponsored by Food Technology found that 50% of them were deficient in Vitamin B6, 42% did not consume enough calcium, 39% had insufficient iron intake, and 25 to 39 percent did not obtain enough vitamin C. One more reason to get a good multi-vitamin in your diet, many people do not realize that they are deficient in nutrients and end up going to the doctor for ailments, ending up on medications instead of simple vitamins.

CHAPTER TEN
FITNESS SUPPLEMENTS

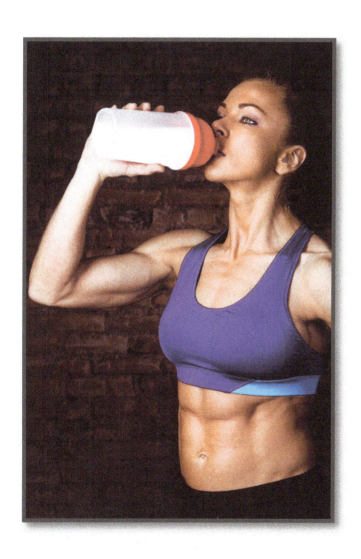

CHAPTER TEN
FITNESS SUPPLEMENTS

Whey Protein Concentrate

This protein is considered to have the highest biological value of any protein source. Whey concentrate is processed the least. It is also the most affordable because of that. A filtering process takes place to remove some of the fats and lactose, retaining a larger protein molecule. Consumers who are not as concerned about a little extra fat or lactose and the percentage of potency of whey feel the concentrate works well for their needs. It is this form of whey that hit the market many years ago as the new best thing, but over the years of new products being introduced, it has been pushed aside as not as good, but it is still a good product. Typically it contains 70-80% protein. Good whey concentrates contain high levels of IGF-1, CLA, Immunoglobins, and Lactoferrins that support the immune system.

Whey Isolate

This form of whey is considered one of the best and is produced similarly to concentrate except the filtration process collects more of the fats and lactose, leaving a higher amount of protein, usually 90% and benefits consumers that can't have lactose and want a pure clean product with easy digestion. Blue Bonnet Nutrition offers an all-natural grass-fed beef form of whey isolate, and ALLMAX Nutrition also offers a good quality whey isolate, one of the few companies that puts a full protein percentage content right on the label and are proud to do so.

Whey Hydrolysate

Make room for the up-and-coming protein. This is one of the newest forms of whey, or at least the latest to get attention in the nutrition health industry. This form of whey goes through enzymatic hydrolysis, a processing method that uses enzymes and water to reduce whey protein molecules into smaller, more digestible proteins and peptides. Whey hydrolysate offers protein absorption and utilization. It is a good choice for consumers with dairy allergies and digestive problems. Now Foods offers a quality hydrolysate whey.

Ion-Exchanged Whey

Here is yet another form of whey protein. It is also a good source, but does lack a few things that you get in the other whey products mentioned above. To put it simply, ion-exchanged whey takes the concentrate whey and processes it through a column for ion-exchange. Due to the processing of ion-exchange whey, some of the good health promoting parts of the whey are depleted or reduced. This makes it a less attractive choice, but many companies still manufacture it this way as their isolate source simply because of the higher protein content. This product will still work for you, but there are other choices out there to consider and compare it to.

Micro-Filtered Whey

This is a whey isolate that is processed using a low temperature cross-flow micro filtration production method. It allows high protein up to 90% availability and maintains important subfractions. This has low fat, low lactose, and no un-denatured proteins. This makes for a non-chemical process and is a good protein choice.

Egg White Protein

This is a good source of protein. The benefits are many, starting with low carbohydrates, contains vitamins, minerals, and all the essential amino acids. Egg whites are a good source of low fat, low carb protein and have been considered a popular and good healthy fitness food for many years.

Casein Protein

A slow-releasing protein shown to help with muscle recovery and growth and even supports immune system health. Casein protein makes up about 80% of cow's milk the other 20% whey. The milk goes through a filtering process to extract the casein. This slow-digesting protein has a great amino acid profile and is often taken just before bed to feed the muscles while you sleep. It can also be taken during the day if it's going to be a long time in between meals. The body will slowly digest the casein protein in some individuals up to seven hours. This is a good choice for individuals who are in heavy training or that are not getting sufficient protein intake during the day.

L-Glutamine

This amino acid is one of the most important supplements to be taken by fitness enthusiasts. L-Glutamine is the most abundant amino acid found in your muscle tissue and plays a key role in the recovery and building of your muscles. An added benefit of this amino acid is that it's known to increase your growth hormone production. 2000 mg. after training and/or before bed is best for optimal results. L-Glutamine has been shown to stop wasting syndrome in people suffering from illness. It also supports a healthy colon.

L-Carnitine

This amino acid is best known for its fat burning properties. Research shows that this supplement has a dramatic effect on fat metabolism. I suggest 1000 mg. 2x day in liquid form on an empty stomach twenty minutes before workout or food. It targets specific stored fat areas while being stimulant free. I recommend Olympia Health brand.

Chitosan

This dietary supplement is a fiber product derived from shellfish. Chitosan absorbs up to twelve times its weight in fat when consumed prior to a fatty meal. This product should be taken apart from fat-soluble vitamins and medications.

Soy Protein

This supplement serves as a very beneficial plant-based meal replacement and dietary supplement. It can be used for fitness goals or just for overall health. And lactose-free soy does contain estrogen properties which can support women's menopause symptoms but must be used with care.

Amino Acids

You may have heard talk about amino acids but never knew exactly what they were. Well, here is a brief summary to help you learn about them. First of all, amino acids are the building blocks of protein. All of the many thousands of proteins found in the human body are made from the twenty essential amino acids. Of these twenty amino acids, the adult body can produce all but eight: Leucine, Lysine, Isoleucine, Methionine,

Phenylalanine, Threonine, Tryptophan and Valine. Now since the body can't produce them, the essential aminos must come from the foods we consume or supplements taken. The necessary amounts of all twenty aminos must be present at the same time to ensure that your body will make the best use of the protein, consume for repair, growth and recovery from your exercise program.

When you take amino acid supplements make sure you consume quality grade, established brands of aminos to achieve the best possible results.

Here are the three groupings of amino acids that you should know:

Branched Chain Amino Acids

Branched chain amino acids are three of the eight essential amino acids whose main function is that of protein synthesis. They are Leucine, Isoleucine and Valine, which are extremely important for recovery and muscle mass stimulation. There has been research that has shown that taking branched chain amino acids within thirty minutes after a workout can help prevent muscle tissue breakdown, increased levels of protein synthesis and prevent muscle catabolism. I consider this not only important for those who work-out trying to increase lean muscle mass. But it is also very important for those persons that may suffer from any diseases that induces muscle wasting and severe weight loss and when combined with L-Glutamine the results will be significantly increased.

Free Form Amino Acids

"Free Form" actually is a meaning for amino acids that are composed of the twenty essential amino acids pooled together without bonds.

These aminos help to keep your body on an "insurance Policy," meaning that your body will have a complete complement of all the aminos when needed. These aminos are best taken on an empty stomach approximately thirty minutes before meals to ensure fast absorption into the bloodstream.

Peptide Bonds

This is a reference to the number of aminos bonded or held together. The two types of Peptide Bonds are Dipeptides and Tripeptides. The meaning of this is "Di" means two aminos bonded together and "Tri" means three or more bonded together. There has always been some controversy around if free form aminos are better than peptide bonds and vice-versa. My opinion is that you will have benefits from either/or and that you should try to consume capsules, powder or liquid aminos rather than those huge horse pills that are dangerous to swallow and not as easy to digest than the aminos in the above mentioned forms.

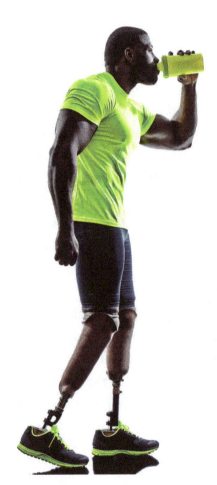

**The power of dedication.
Let nothing stop you from your dreams!**

Here are some of the best finds for workout supplements and overall sense of well-being. It doesn't matter what level of working out you're at, there is something good to pick from for everyone's needs.

D-aspartic acid

This is a great product for anyone looking to add strength and lean muscle size. It will also increase the sperm count and keep you very fertile for those who want it. This supplement has been said to increase natural testosterone levels up to forty-percent in a relatively short period of time. Our feed back on this product at my nutrition center is excellent and I have taken this myself and like it. Three grams per day must be taken to achieve proper results either with the first meal of the day or in a pre-workout supplement. In the Italian research studies a dozen men were given three grams per day and after 12 days their testosterone was up forty-two percent compared to the placebo group. This natural amino acid shows promising results for the fitness industry.

VPX - NO Shotgun

This original formula is one of the best pre-workout supplements on the market. I personally take this myself. Just take one scoop mixed in water thirty minutes before you work out on an empty stomach. It is one of the few pre-workouts that give you protein, nitric oxide, BCAAs, L-Glutamine, and much more. You will get energy that will last through your workout and pump you up, give you great strength, and just enough caffeine to get you going but not make you over-stimulated. This is the original formula you need to ask for. There is also a stimulant-free version available for those of you that can't take stimulants, called Synthesize, also by VPX. You will love this product and I tell you what I feel is the truth on all supplements. I have no ties with any of these companies other than retailing the products and getting the feedback on them.

Amino Energy

By ON Nutrition, this is a very good pre-workout supplement. Mild yet effective for both men and women. It will give you just what you need for a good workout and boost, while supplying your amino acids for your repair and recovery from training. This is a top seller since it fits into most lifestyles of training, from beginner to advanced. There is always good feedback from customers on Amino Energy.

Manimal

Power packed. Chaparral Labs in their advertising, says it will make you a gorilla in the gym. This product is a great blend of natural-testosterone producing ingredients. This has all the best of the best, working together to give you energy, strength, endurance, lean muscle mass, libido, and more. It is pro-hormone-free, steroid-free, and contains many ingredients including, Arginine, Tribulus, Muira Puama and more. It is taken three times a day and can even be used as a post cycle after using pro-hormones, or taken right along with them to avoid testosterone shutdown. This is a good product all in one bottle.

* As with all products mentioned, you will need to start with a smaller dosage and work up to what your body, health status, and lifestyle will tolerate. Add D-aspartic acid for great results.

Tribulus

This is a popular herbal supplement that makes you produce more natural testosterone. Many men feel this gives them just enough of a boost in and out of the gym. Tribex is a good formula, as is the extract in capsules from Solaray.

Velvet Deer Antler

You may have recently heard of this one since it has been on the news due to the pro athletes using it as one of their all-natural supplements. It contains a range of growth factors including the metabolite of HGH that is IGH-1. This product has been shown to increase energy, -recovery, endurance, fat loss, muscle mass gain, anti-aging, libido, and immune system support. Pure Factors provides an extra strength formula for athletes and fitness enthusiasts, considered one of the best on the market, and the Now brand offers a good one as well. Antler-Test by Nutra Key is excellent.

A-HD

Bpi brand. This product is a very good anti-estrogen and natural testosterone booster. It gives good results in the gym and is a mild supplement and in most cases safe to use. This can also be taken as a post cycle after doing pro-hormones or other testosterone boosting products. Users often find this product getting them lean muscle mass and good strength gains in the gym.

CLA

Tonalin is the best source and most widely studied. If taken at 3,000 mg. per day, one pill three times a day, studies have shown this to burn fat and increase muscle even without exercise. This is a good product to combine with L-Carnitine for those of you that do not want stimulants in your diet products and want to lose weight steadily and gently. When combined with a good diet and moderate exercise program, many have done well on this product, but this is something you want to take for eight to twelve weeks. It is a steady weight loss, not a quick-fix diet pill.

DHEA

Known as the anti-aging supplement, this hormone is produced in our bodies. It controls the estrogen in women and the testosterone in men, then starts to decline beginning in our mid 20's, and hits a major decline in our 40's, sending women into menopause and men into andropause.

DHEA used to be on prescription years ago and now is available in health food stores and nutrition centers. This product works well when a good quality is purchased. I recommend Douglas Labs as one of the best sources. It is advised that women take 25 mg. per day and men 50 mg. per day. At these low levels, they work well and the body will recognize this hormone as a non-foreign substance since it is used to having it in the body already and will tolerate it well. Do not exceed 100 mg. per day, as that is when side effects can happen. In low dosages for people over forty, this seems to be a safe choice for persons in good health that are looking to turn back the clock some and feel more youthful. DHEA will raise the metabolism to burn fat, increase lean muscle, help with age-related memory issues, tighten the skin, improve heart health, work on fighting inflammation, libido, energy, improve the immune system, fight osteoporosis, and much more. For those of you that do not want to take a hormone product, you can take 7-Keto DHEA which is the non-hormone form.

Green Coffee Bean Extract

Dieting is made a bit easier with this product which was brought to many people's attention on a popular doctor's talk show. This product is known for fighting fat around the mid-section and it must contain GCA and at least 50% chlorogenic acid. Taking two capsules per day at 800 mg. each, one in the morning prior to food and the other mid-afternoon, has given results of two to three pounds of fat loss per week. The feedback from my customers has been good and this product is very well tolerated and is considered mild for most consumers.

Garcinia Cambogia Extract

This popular product is used as a diet appetite suppressant. It has been around for years, but was recently mentioned on a popular doctor's talk show, as was the other one, and it has gotten major attention now. This product contains HCA - hydroxicitric acid, and it must contain at least 50% HCA to be effective. It blocks fats and sugars while reducing appetite, which prevents the formation of fat cells in the body, helping you lose weight. It is suggested to take a pill in the morning prior to food and another in the mid-afternoon.

Testo Extreme

This product is a special formulation and is a good decent balancing formula for men by Olympia Health. It provides a nice testosterone boost, energy, libido, increased metabolism for calorie burning, will help to increase lean muscle with exercise, and creates a better mood and sense of well-being for the user. This product gets built up in the system over the first few weeks of using it and you will feel its full potential after the first bottle. This is a mild yet effective product for a natural testosterone and energy boost and works well combined with the Mega Food Multi-Vitamin for men. Adding a basic workout routine will greatly enhance the effects and you will notice a more productive day whether you work out or not. It is a good choice and the feedback by most men on this product is great.

CHAPTER ELEVEN
NUTRITION, FOOD, AND DIET PLANS

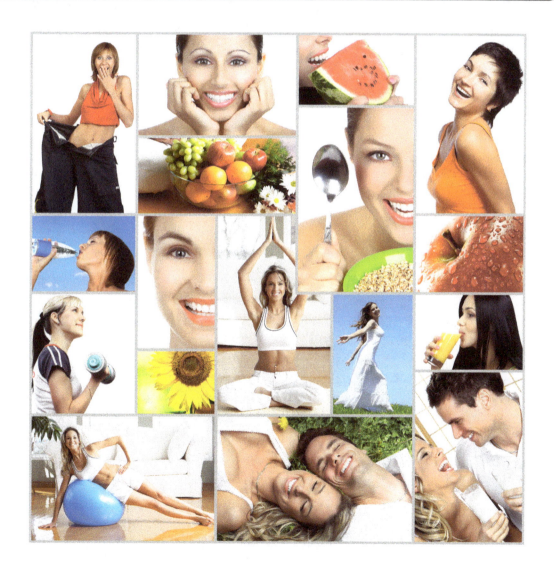

BURN THE FAT FOODS QUICK REFERENCE

LEAN PROTEINS

Food Item	Qty	Calories	Protein	Carbs	Fat
Chicken breast, skinless	4 oz	196	35.1	0	5.1
Beef, ground 96% lean	4 oz	171	28.5	0	5.1
Beef, top sirloin	4 oz	229	34.4	0	9.1
Beef, top round	4 oz	214	35.9	0	6.7
Buffalo, top round	4 oz	195	32.0	0	6.8
Cod	4 oz	119	25.9	0	1.0
Egg whites	6	102	21	1.8	0.0
Egg, whole	1	75	6.3	0.6	5.0
Lobster	4 oz	111	23.2	1.5	0.7
Protein Powder, Whey	2 scoops	180	35	4	3.0
Salmon, Atlantic	4 oz	206	28.8	0	9.2
Shrimp	4 oz	120	23	1	2.0
Tuna, canned in water	4 oz	120	26	0	1.0
Turkey Breast, skinless	4 oz	178	33.9	0	3.7
Turkey, ground 99% lean	4 oz	120	28	0	1.0
Venison steak	4 oz	173	35	0	2.3

COMPLEX CARBS (Starches & Grain)

Food Item	Qty	Calories	Protein	Carbs	Fat
Bagel, plain, whole wheat	1	150	6	33	1
Beans, kidney	1/3 C ckd	75	5.1	13.5	0.3
Bread, whole wheat	1 slice	80	2.5	14	1
Bread, rye	1 slice	80	3	16	1
Potato, white	1 lg (8 oz)	210	4.4	49	0.2
Potato, sweet	4 oz	136	2.1	31.6	0.4
Oatmeal, old-fashioned	1/3 C unckd	100	5	16	2
Cream of Rice	1/4 C unckd	170	3	38	0
Cream of Wheat	1 oz/1 pckt	100	3	21	1
Lentils	1/2 C ckd	115	9	20	0
Black-eyed peas	1/2 C boiled	99	6.6	17.7	0.4
Pita, whole wheat	1	170	6	35	2
Pasta, whole grain spelt	1 oz (dry)	95	4	20	0.7
Pasta, whole wheat	1 oz (dry)	105	4.5	20	1
Rice, brown ("Success")	1 C ckd	150	4	40	0
Rice, wild	1 C ckd	166	6.5	35	0.6
Kashi cereal	3/4 cup	120	8	28	1
Shredded Wheat	1 cup	144	3.6	33.4	1.4
Yam	6 oz	180	4	41	0.2

BURN THE FAT FOODS QUICK REFERENCE

DAIRY PRODUCTS

Food Item	Qty	Calories	Protein	Carbs	Fat
Milk, skim	1 cup	90	8	12	1
Milk, 1% lowfat	1 cup	100	8	11	2
Cheese, American, nonfat	2 slices	80	12	6	0
Cheese, Cheddar	1 oz	114	7	9	1
Cheese, Mozzarella, nonfat	1/2 cup	90	18	4	0
Cheese, Parmesan, nonfat	2 tbsp	75	10	10	0
Cottage cheese, nonfat	5 oz	100	17.5	5	1.3
Cottage cheese, 2% lowfat	1/2 cup	103	15.5	4	2
Cottage cheese, 1% lowfat	5 oz	100	17.5	5	1.3
Cottage cheese, nonfat	5 oz	100	16.2	7.5	0
Sour cream, nonfat	2 tbsp	20	2.5	2.5	0
Yogurt, nonfat	8 oz (1)	100	8	17	0
Yogurt, fruit, 1% lowfat	8 oz (1)	250	9	50	2
Yogurt, froz, nonfat, no sug	1 cup	160	8	38	0

FRUIT (Natural Simple Carbs)

Food Item	Qty	Calories	Protein	Carbs	Fat
Apples	1	81	0.3	21.1	0.5
Banana	1	105	1.2	26.7	0.6
Blueberries	1 cup	82	1.0	20.4	0.6
Cantaloupe	1/2	94	2.3	22.3	0.7
Grapefruit	1/2	46	0.6	11.9	0.1
Grapes (seedless)	10	36	0.3	8.9	0.3
Jelly, all fruit (no sugar)	2 tbsp	80	0	20	0
Nectarine	1	67	1.3	16	0.6
Orange	1	65	1.4	16.3	0.1
Peach	1	37	0.6	9.7	0.1
Pear	1	98	0.7	25.1	0.7
Plum	1	36	0.5	8.6	0.4
Raisins	1/4 cup	130	1.0	31	0.5
Raspberries	1 cup	62	1.2	14.2	0.6
Strawberries	1 cup	46	1.0	10.4	0.6
Watermelon (diced)	1 cup	50	1.0	3.6	0.2

BURN THE FAT FOODS QUICK REFERENCE

FIBROUS CARBS (Veggies & Greens)

Food Item	Qty	Calories	Protein	Carbs	Fat
Asparagus	10 spears	40	4	6	0
Broccoli	1 cup	46	4.6	8.6	0.4
Brussels sprouts	1 cup	60	4	11.6	0.4
Cauliflower	1 cup	60	4.8	13.6	0.8
Carrots	1	31	0.8	7.3	0.1
Collard Greens	2 cups	36	1.6	8	0.4
Corn	1/2 cup	89	2.7	20.6	1.1
Cucumber	1 cup	16	0.6	3	0.2
Green pepper	1 cup	24	0	6	0
Green beans	6 oz	50	2	12	0
Kale	2 cups	56	4	11.6	0.8
Lettuce	2 cups	20	0	6	0
Onion	1 cup	54	2	12	0
Mushrooms	1 C ckd	42	3.4	8	0.8
Peas	1/2 cup	57	4	10	0
Salsa	4 tbsp	16	0	4	0
Spinach	1 C ckd	42	5.4	6.8	0.4
Tomato	1 med	24	1	5	0
Zucchini	1 cup	16	1.4	3.2	0.2

FATS, OILS, NUTS & SEEDS

Food Item	Qty	Calories	Protein	Carbs	Fat
Avocado	1 med	115	3	9	15
Almonds	1 oz	170	6	5	15
Cashews	1/2 cup	394	10.5	22.4	31.7
Canola oil	1 tbsp	120	0	0	14
Flaxseed oil	1 tbsp	130	0	0	14
Flaxseed, ground	1 oz	151	5	8	12
Peanuts	1/2 cup	428	17.3	15.7	36.3
Peanut butter, natural	1 tbsp	100	3.5	3.5	8
Olive oil	1 tbsp	120	0	0	13.6
Udo's essential oil blend	1 tbsp	134	0	0	14.2
Salad dressing, Italian	1 tbsp	82	0	2	9
Salad dressing, Olive & Vngr	1 tbsp	75	0	0.5	8
Salad dressing, Light Italian	3 tbsp	12	0	3	0
Walnuts	1 oz	200	5	3	20

Good and Bad Fats

There is always controversy around fats. Many times people think they are to avoid all fats, and when they see fats listed on the labels, they put the product down. But the truth of the matter is that we need fats, good fats, to support our everyday body functions and keep us in good health.

Monounsaturated fats and polyunsaturated fats are the "Good Fats". They are good for your heart, lowering cholesterol, good for brain function, bodily functions, skin, hair, and overall health. You will find these good fats in such foods as salmon, tuna, sardines, flaxseeds, sunflower seeds, sesame seeds, almonds, cashews, peanut butter, avocados, soymilk, safflower oil, and olive oil.

Saturated fats and trans fats are the "Bad Fats". They tend to be solid at room temperature such as margarine and shortening. Be sure to avoid fried foods like French fries and fried chicken. You will also find these bad fats in many candy bars, commercially baked cookies, pastries, and several pre-packaged snack foods. Make sure you remove the skin from your chicken before cooking it, try to eat less red meat, this includes pork, and eat more fish and chicken. Always bake or grill your foods and use Olive Oil or Canola Oil in your cooking. Keep dairy products to a minimum and purchase them in low fat forms.

Omega 3 fish oils and Flaxseed oils are really good to have as a regular daily intake. Make sure the Omega 3 fish oil is distilled and mercury free and that the Flax oil is cold pressed and organic. What we eat contributes to our "good" cholesterol (HDL) and our "bad" cholesterol (LDL).

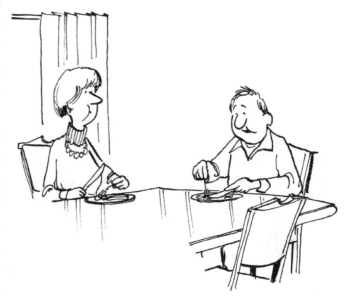

"Ooo, I just felt the good cholesterol kick the bad cholesterol."

Daily Basics

Lesson 1

Keep a daily log in a small notebook, or on the charts I've provided, of what you're eating and drinking throughout the day. This way you'll be able to review what you've written and this alone will help you control your eating habits just because you will start to relate everything you go to put in your mouth with the accountability of having to write it down and this makes you less likely to cheat.

Lesson 2

Look at the Fat grams, Carbohydrates and Sugar content of the foods you are eating. Just because it says "Fat Free" doesn't mean it's okay to eat especially if it is high in sugar grams which will eventually be converted and stored as a fat especially the closer it is to bedtime. Try to keep your carb intake lower as the day goes on.

Lesson 3

After 6 pm and/or 4 to 5 hours prior to going to bed for your night's rest, consume NO bread, white rice, pasta, corn or potatoes, NO fruit or fruit juices, and drink only a good bottled water with a lemon wedge or tea sweetened only with Stevia.

Lesson 4

Eat a balance of smaller meals that consist of green salads and vegetables (no Corn), water-packed Tuna, Turkey Breast (low salt), baked or broiled Chicken Breast, and baked Fish. If you do not have time to prepare one of these meals, then you may substitute with a Protein Shake or High Protein / Low Carb Bar.

Lesson 5

No soft drinks and only consume beverages that are sweetened with natural sweeteners. I do not like to see a lot of aspartame type products being consumed and if you do feel the need to consume these types of products then please make sure to keep it to a minimum. Try to drink 6-8 large glasses of bottled water per day, I recommend distilled water since it will remove the most impurities from your system, or a good pH balanced water that will provide oxygen to the body.

Lesson 6

Consume no fried foods and use no products that have hydrogenated oils in them since this will be very poor health wise for your body especially your cardiovascular system. Consume NO fast food since these products are loaded for the most part with high fat and salt. Once your body tastes these high sodium products they will start to crave salt and it can become addictive to the point where your body will start sending signals to your brain for more salt which will in turn make you think that your craving another fast food meal that you thought was so good, but in fact it's just your body wanting a quick fix for some more salty fries almost like what happens to an alcoholic with liquor but in this case it's foods high in sodium and fats. Once you break away from this bad habit you'll see your body will not want this type of food anymore and what you once thought was good will actually not taste all that great anymore and you'll feel a lot better because of it. Your body is supposed to get recharged and energized from the foods we consume, yet so many people eat the wrong foods and feel like going to sleep afterwards because these fast foods put a major strain on our bodies and digestive tracts.

STAY AWAY FROM THESE FOODS – Start to listen to your body and how you feel afterwards. Our bodies are set up to take the nutrition from the foods we consume and turn it into an energy source to feed our bodies and build our cells for over-all health. Listen to your body and you will find that it will speak to you about its needs, however this will only start to happen after about two weeks of good eating habits after your body has started to cleanse itself from all the sugar, salt and high fat foods that so many people consume. Try opening the gas tank of your car and throw a cup of sugar and salt down it, you know what would happen? It would ruin your car engine beyond repair, a car that most people would only expect to last ten years anyway, yet when it come to our bodies that are expected to last a whole lifetime, people throw all this sugar and salt down their throat and into their bodies and still expect their internal human engines to run without any problems, well this just isn't the case and the time is now to make these changes for a better YOU!

Lesson 7

1. Park your car in the furthest parking space NOT the closest.
2. Take the stairs whenever possible not the elevator, and if you have to go up several stories then get off two floors sooner and walk up the last 2 flights.
3. Walk some place for lunch instead of driving if there is a place close by.
4. Get off the bus one or two blocks further from work or home.
5. Give yourself a "cheat day" one day per week when you can eat anything you want within reason. This will help you to stick to your routine the rest of the week. The one cheat meal will not hurt you; it's the every day cheats that end up getting you in the long run.

These tips may not seem like much, but by the end of the month they add up. As an example: the person that decides to get off the elevator 2 flights sooner, this will add up to 6 flights per day if you count lunch, which will add up to 120 flights of steps per month that you would have climbed or 1440 flights per year figured on a five day work week. You see there is always ways to exercise even when we think there's no time. Where there's a will there's a way!! As the popular saying goes, "Whether you think you can or think you can't, you're right."

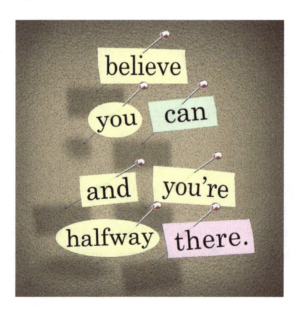

SAMPLE DIET #1

Healthy & Fit Daily Diet Plan

Good for everyone to follow as a guide 6 days a week

MEAL 1 7:00 a.m. Breakfast	Whey or Soy protein shake mixed with juice or low fat milk and a banana. – or – Bowl of Oatmeal with low fat milk 3 egg whites hard boiled spray pan with olive oil Coffee / tea plain or with Stevia sweetener
MEAL 2 10:00 a.m. Snack	Protein Bar – low sugar / low carb – or – Greek yogurt low sugar / high protein
MEAL 3 12:30 p.m. Lunch	1 can water-packed Tuna with Lemon juice, Olive oil over lettuce with carrots, tomato. – or – 1 small skinless Chicken Breast (baked, broiled, grilled) and ½ cup brown rice, small salad (vinegar / oil)
MEAL 4 3:00 p.m. Midday Snack	High protein, low carb bar or protein shake and tablespoon of flaxseed oil
MEAL 5 6:00 p.m. Dinner	1 portion (4-6 ounces) of Chicken Breast, Fish or Lean Beef (grilled, broiled, baked) and green vegetable, bottled water
MEAL 6 8:30 p.m. Snack	1 scoop protein powder (low carb) 2 frozen strawberries, Ice, 6 oz skim milk or water, blend into pudding consistency. – or – Low carb protein bar

Note: For those that need to gain weight, a high calorie weight gain shake can be substituted for the low carb shakes.

David Anthony's Make Me Skinny Diet
Low Calorie Weight Loss Plan
(Followed 6 days a week)

Meal #1 Breakfast	Whey Isolate Protein Shake (1 scoop) mixed in water (110 calories) One Bitter-Orange Standarized Extract Cap with 1 tbsp liquid L-Carnitine 30 minutes before shake One Tonalin CLA softgel 1,000mg with shake.
Meal #2 Mid-AM snack	Quest Bar
Meal #3 Lunch	3.5 oz. Chicken Breast, baked (173 calories) 1/2 cup Brown Rice (108 calories) 1 cup Green Beans (46 calories) Water
Meal #4 Mid-PM snack	Whey Isolate Protein Shake (1 scoop) (117 calories) mixed in water with 2 strawberries/ice. 1 Bitter-Orange Standarized Extract Cap 30 minutes before shake 1 tbsp liquid L-Carnitine 30 minutes before shake. One Tonalin CLA softgel 1,000mg with shake.
Meal #5 Dinner	3 oz. Salmon, baked (151 calories) 1 serving Broccoli (4 florets) (30 calories) One Tonalin CLA softgel 1,000mg with dinner. One mega hoodia capsule 30 min before dinner. Water
Meal #6 PM snack (optional)	5 oz. Cottage Cheese, 1% low fat (100 calories) 1 oz. Almonds, raw, mixed with 1 tbsp flaxseed oil sprinkled with cinnamon

Lean Muscle Diet

(Followed 6 days a week)

Meal #1 Breakfast	5-6 Egg Whites, cooked 1 cup Oatmeal, cooked Water (Liq L-Carnitine 20 min before food)
Meal #2 Mid-AM snack	Whey Isolate Protein Shake (1-2 scoops) mixed in low fat 1% milk or water with 1/2 banana 1 food based multi-vitamin/mineral tablet
Meal #3 Lunch	1 can Tuna in water or Baked Fish 1 small salad, Lettuce with low cal dressing (2 tbsp) 2 hard-boiled Eggs Water
Meal #4 Mid-PM snack	Whey Isolate Protein Shake (1-2 scoops) mixed in low fat 1% milk or water
Meal #5 Dinner	4 oz. Salmon or Chicken Breast, baked or grilled 1 cup Green Beans 1/2 cup Brown Rice Water
Meal #6 PM snack	5 oz. Cottage Cheese, 1% low fat (100 calories) 1 oz. Almonds, raw, mixed with 1 tbsp flaxseed oil sprinkled with cinnamon

*Note: On day 7 you may add a cheat meal of choice to any of the 6 day per week diet plans.

Bulk Up Diet
Adding Size for Hard Gainers

Weight gain supplements that get good results and positive feedback:
* MHP Up Your Mass   * Optimum Serious Mass   * Real Gains
* Arnold Mass   * Cyto-Gainer from Cyto Sport   * Dymatize Mass

Meal #1
Breakfast
	5-6 Eggs (2 yolks)
	3.5 oz. Lean Beef or Chicken, broiled or grilled
	1 cup Oatmeal, cooked
	Universal Animal Pak (30 min. after your meal) -
	  If a workout day, take Animal Pak 30 min. after
	  the meal that's prior to your workout.
	Water and digestive enzyme.

Meal #2 Mid-AM snack	1 Weight Gain shake (Pick from above listing) 1 tsp Micronized Creatine mixed into shake 1 tbsp Flaxseed Oil
Meal #3 Lunch	4 oz Chicken Breast or Lean Beef, baked. 1 Sweet Potato 1 cup Green Beans Water
Workout (wait 2 hours After last meal.)	Pre-workout Supplement (workout days only) 1 scoop VPX NO - Shotgun mixed in water 30 minutes before workout. Post-workout Supplement - Take 1 heaping tsp Micronized Creatine powder in grape juice immediately following workout, wait 30 minutes and have Meal #4 shake listed below.
Meal #4 Mid-PM snack	1 Weight Gain shake 1 Banana
Meal #5 Dinner	8 oz. Sirloin Steak 1 cup Brown Rice 1 cup Broccoli, Water and digestive enzyme.
Meal # 6	1 Weight Gain shake (before bed)

Ultimate Fat Burner Diet

Two days before starting diet take the 48 Hour Cleanse by Solaray.

Meal #1)   Whey Protein Isolate Shake in water one scoop
One Whole Food Multi Vitamin
One tablespoon Liquid L-Carnitine
One Hydroxi-Elite Capsule by Hi- Tech Pharm

Meal #2)   One Quest Protein Bar, bottle of water / unsweet tea

Meal #3)   Water Packed Tuna (drained) over bed of lettuce
With chopped carrots and tomato sprinkle
Lemon juice, olive oil and vinegar with a little
Pepper if wanted and bottle of water.
(may have 3.5oz grilled chicken on top of lettuce instead)

Meal #4)   Whey Protein Isolate Shake one scoop
One tablespoon Flax Oil
One Hydroxi –Elite Capsule by Hi-Tech Pharm.

Meal #5)   Grilled or baked Salmon or Chicken(skinless) 3.5oz
Green Beans –Steamed.
One mega hoodia capsule 30 min before dinner
Water

Meal #6)   Celery and Carrot Sticks,
10 Raw Almonds.

Note: You must be in good health to do this diet. The Hydroxi- Elite has a stimulant in it, you may want to start your first day with just one pill to get used to your tolerance and go up to the 2nd pill in afternoon when you feel ready. Discontinue immediately if you feel any side effects.

Week _____

DAYS	FOODS CONSUMED Breakfast-Snack-Lunch-Snack-Dinner-Snack
Sunday	
Monday	
Tuesday	
Wednesday	
Thursday	
Friday	
Saturday	

Comments:

* Make copies of this page to track your meals.
* Note that you will still take your supplements on your 7th day, but you can add your cheat meal in.

CHAPTER TWELVE
NUTRITION AND THE BIBLE

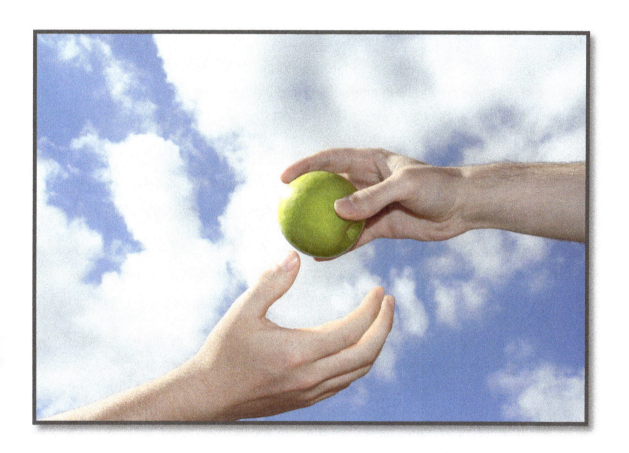

CHAPTER TWELVE
NUTRITION AND THE BIBLE

What the Bible says we should eat

So many times in this modern day and age, as the alternative treatment popularity has expanded with herbal remedies and various other natural treatments, and so forth, we often hear someone talk about this latest "fad" and how it's possible that this new "wonder" product is just a scheme to get your money and how these products "won't" work or some shows actually have someone from the pharmaceutical industry to downplay the results or even a physician not trained in natural medicine to "scare" you into not trying these new natural alternative products.

Well, my friends, the fact of the matter is that the natural remedies have an ancient history behind them and have been around far longer than modern day medicine.

In fact, several health tips are found right in the Bible.

I believe God put everything we need and will ever need right here on this earth.

Alternative care through natural medicine can be used to a large extent to actually prevent a lot of health problems that you would eventually end up needing surgery for. An example of this would be keeping cholesterol levels low in the body so you would not ever need bypass surgery which is very common in today's conventional medicine. We all know someone or have heard of someone that has had a bypass surgery.

I like to see people actually prevent disease through lifestyle change.

God wants us to be healthy. But due to the human race being given "self will," we make our own decisions about how to take care of our bodies through our diets and exercise programs. However, God promises us eternal life for our souls not our bodies, so the physical body part is up to us. Even so, when a person gets ill they often ask why God let this happen to them. God gave them free will, they often in some cases, may have done this to themselves by lack of proper diet and exercise and some bad habits.

Our modern day processed foods, harsh chemicals in everything from our foods and drinking water to our air and beauty supplies and various other items that we come in daily contact with, most of them are driven by financial gain and not by the common good for our people. These items continue to put toxicity into our food sources and our bodies and it is up to us to cleanse ourselves and supplement to counter act these harmful invaders that slowly creep into our healthy bodies.

Knowledge is the key. Take the time to read labels and make as many things homemade as you can or buy them with the least amount of preservatives and chemicals possible.

There is a time and place for modern medicine in our lives but let us never forget who the real physician is.

I remember standing in my store one day and a lady was talking about how wonderful this doctor was whom she took her son to at the emergency room when he broke his arm in two places. The doctor set it in a cast that her son had to wear for several weeks and when the cast came off he regained full use of his arm.

She went on to say that the doctor "healed" her son's arm and that it was as good as new and that this doctor had performed a "miracle" because with the multiple breaks that her son had, he should have not regained full use of his arm.

Yes, the doctor did put it in the cast, it is important to have a good doctor which many times God works through, but God knitted the bone and skin back together with this incredible body he gave us that is capable of performing miracles every day. But they are often overlooked by many. Our God given gift to heal itself, and in a way, we all have super hero powers. Many times we underestimate our own bodies' capabilities. It is time to own the decisions you make for your body and make better daily choices for your health.

Here are some health tips from the Bible

Psalms 103:2

> "Praise the Lord, O my soul, and forget not all his benefits, who forgives all your sins and heals all your diseases."

All God's people began as vegetarians, yet after the Great Flood God gave his permission to us to eat some types of meat.

Leviticus 11:2-3

> "These are the beasts which ye shall eat among all the beasts that are on the earth. Whatsoever parteth the hoof, and is cloven footed and cheweth the cud, among the beasts, that shall ye eat."

Toxins are known to be higher as you move up the food chain. Meat-eating creatures have more poisons than vegetarian creatures. God told his people to eat vegetarian animals that thoroughly chew their food and have multi-chambered stomachs. These animals have a much lower risk of disease, infections and parasites.

Cows, chickens, turkeys and sheep that were all fed vegetarian diets in Moses' day were all allowed under God's law. Now on the other hand, pigs (pork) do not chew their foods and they eat just about anything they can get, which opens them up to carry infections and worms. Chicken and turkey are high in protein while being low in fat and sheep are known for their rich omega- 3's.

Now we are also given guidelines on the type of fish to eat.

Leviticus 11:9

> "These shall ye eat of all that are in the waters whatsoever hath fins and scales in the seas, and in the rivers, them shall ye eat."

Here we are told to eat fish with fins and scales such as salmon, haddock, sole, and tuna. These fish are clean and build the immune system. We should not eat shellfish such as shrimp, lobster and clams since they are more of a filter fish class and gather more poisons. *(Several references are made in Leviticus about foods. I suggest you read it in its entirety.)

Deuteronomy 8:8

"A land with wheat and barley, vines and fig trees, pomegranates; olive oil and honey."

Jesus was known for eating barley bread. Barley is rich in tocotrienols, which is a substance similar, yet believed to be stronger than Vitamin E, which helps lower the risk of heart disease.

Genesis 1:30

"And to all the beasts of the earth and all the birds of the air and all the creatures that move on the ground - everything that has the breath of life in it - I give every green plant for food."

God knew how important our vegetables would be to our health. Carrots for their carotenoids and bioflavanoids, which help as free radical protectors, help as immune boosters and even slow down aging.

Cruciferous vegetables like broccoli, which helps lower the risk of cancer and provides the body with vital nutritional and energizing properties that help heal and build the immune system.

Numbers 11:5

"We remember the fish, which we did eat in Egypt freely; the cucumbers and the melons, and the leeks, and the onions and the garlic."

Garlic is considered to have antibiotic properties. It has been shown to lower blood pressure, cleanse the blood, boost the immune system against disease and infections, lower cholesterol and help improve overall health.

Song of Solomon 2:5

> "Comfort me with apples."

You may have heard the saying "an apple a day keeps the doc away." Well, apples are rich in fiber and can help cleanse the colon, while lowering cholesterol in the blood and cleansing your teeth. Apple cider vinegar has been shown to have several benefits including helping with arthritis, weight loss, parasite cleansing and much more.

Isaiah 7:15, 22

> "He will eat curds and honey when he knows enough to refuse the evil and choose the good."

This butter or curd type product is believed by many to refer to yogurt, which contains acidophilus which is known to put friendly bacteria into your intestinal wall, which boosts the immune system and helps fight infection.

Honey has bioflavonoids and antibiotic properties to prevent infections and is a healthy natural sweetener with some additional anti-allergy properties to the outdoors. It's been known to help with hay fever if you get the honey from a local bee keeper and as long as you're not allergic to bee stings.

Ezekiel 4:9

> "Take thou also unto thee wheat and barley, beans and lentils, millet and fitches; put them in a vessel jar and use them to make bread thereof."

Now what this actually means is that these types of proteins complement each other and are often well tolerated by the body. You can actually find Ezekiel bread at your local health food store.

Legumes, meaning beans, are high in protein and really go a long way, so they are quite affordable and nutritious especially for the poor. Soybeans contain genistein, which has been shown to have health benefits.

Mark 6:41

"Taking the five loaves and the two fish and looking up to heaven, he gave thanks and broke the loaves."

Luke 5:4,6

"And the Lord said "Launch out into the deep, and let down your nets for a draught. And when they had this done, they enclosed a great multitude of fishes."

Fish is high in protein, mostly low in fat, and the fats that they do contain are "good fats." These are your omega-3 oils shown to help fight cancer and heart disease. These EPA oils also help with arthritis as anti-inflammatories; they feed the brain for nerve function, and are rich in B-6 and selenium.

Fish is very important to one's health when prepared properly and when consumed on a regular basis can have great benefits.

The sign of the fish is often used as a symbol of one's Christianity.

Mark 12:30, 31

"Love the Lord thy God with all thy heart and thou shalt love thy neighbor as thyself, there is none other commandments greater than these."

John 6:54

"Whoso eateth my flesh, and drinketh my blood, hath eternal life; and I will raise him up at the last day."

Luke 6:37

"Judge not, and ye shall not be judged: condemn not, and ye shall not be condemned: forgive, and ye shall be forgiven."

John 3:15

"That whosoever believeth in him should not perish, but have eternal life."

CHAPTER THIRTEEN
WHAT'S IN YOUR FOOD?

Toxic ingredients you should know about

As you're taking supplements and beverages throughout your day, there are some toxins in products that you need to be aware of and avoid. Try to consume organic meats, fruits and vegetables, and supplements whenever possible.

BVO

This can be found in many beverages. It prevents the flavoring from floating to the top so it doesn't have to be shaken before use. Many countries have banned BVO but it is still allowed in the U.S. It has been linked to some thyroid diseases, cancer, and auto-immune diseases. Brominated vegetable oil.

Coloring Agents

Blue 1, Blue 2, Yellow 5, Yellow 6. These colors are made from coal tar that is used to kill bugs and to wax and shine floors, and can be toxic in high consumption.

BHA / BHT

These are found in some cereals, nut mixes, gum, butter, meats, and beer to name a few. BHA/BHT are made from petroleum and act as a preservative. They are known to have possible cancer causing effects since it is a carcinogen.

RBGH / BBST

These are synthetic hormones given to cows and are passed into their milk and their meat. In some cases, it has been linked to breast cancer, prostate cancer, and infertility.

Arsenic

This toxic substance has been found in some chicken feed to produce "pinker" meat, and can cause sickness in humans.

Propylene glycol alginate (E405)

This is used as a food thickener and stabilizer. It is also used as an emulsifier and is derived from algenic acid esterfied and combined with propylene glycol. Now even though propylene glycol is used as a food additive, it is also a popular industrial product used in automobile antifreezes and airport runway de-icers during winter months.

Polysorbate 60

Polyoxyethylene (20) sorbitan monostearate. This is an emulsifier popular in the food industry. It is made of corn, palm oil, and petroleum. This mix won't spoil, so it's often used to replace dairy in baked goods and liquid products.

MSG

Monosodium glutamate, a flavor enhancer found in many products. FDA approved. Can, in some cases, cause symptoms of learning disabilities, Parkinson's disease, neurological diseases, obesity, disorientation, eye problems, numbness, drowsiness, headaches, and weakness.

Aspartame

This substance is considered by many to be the most dangerous substance on the market today. It is also called Equal and NutraSweet. It accounts for 75% of all adverse side effects in food additives. So many take this substance to help slim down, but the truth is hardly anyone ever loses weight. Some studies show Aspartame to be linked to headaches, joint pain, aches, cancer, insomnia, Type 2 diabetes, heart problems, tumors, depression, and so on. It is used in beverages, supplements, gum, and baked goods. The FDA still labels this product as safe, but many studies and cases tell a different story. At 95 degrees, the artificial sweetener actually turns to formaldehyde. (The human body is 98.6 degrees.)

Red #40

This is the most widely used and consumed dye. It may accelerate the appearance of tumors in mice. It also causes allergy-like symptoms in consumers and might trigger hyperactivity in children.

Sodium Nitrate

This is a salt that is used as a preservative, especially in lunch meats and pre-packaged bacon, hot dogs, hams, and various other products. It is said that it can lead to the cancer-causing molecules that can result in tumor formation, and that it can move across the placenta. Nitrates have been linked to cancer through the production of nitrosamines, according to the Linus Pauling Institute. It is good to avoid the products that contain this ingredient. If you do consume it, take extra Vitamin C which is said to help balance out some of the negative side effects. It also can give you a stiffness in your body after a couple days of consumption, so limit your intake.

Toxic food ingredients just might make you look and feel different, you may just not feel like yourself. Always think twice before you consume ingredients you're not familiar with and make sure you read labels and ask questions.

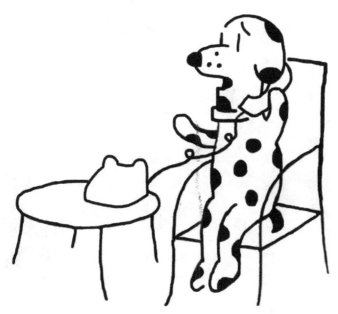

"That's just the problem, Doctor.
I'm not a Dalmation."

CHAPTER FOURTEEN
AROMATHERAPY FOR BALANCE OF HEALTH

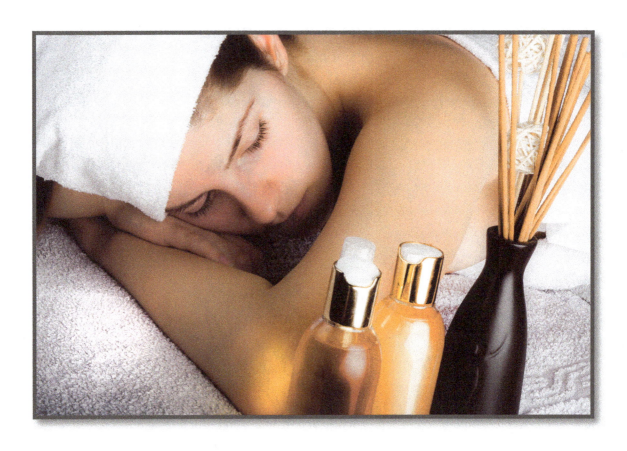

CHAPTER FOURTEEN
AROMATHERAPY FOR BALANCE OF HEALTH

APPLICATION OF THE OILS

Most everyone can benefit from the use of essential oils. Whether you inhale essential scents each afternoon for a quick energy boost, or relax in a soothing tub before bedtime, the oils can be used throughout the day to help with stress and to increase energy. You can place a small dab on your skin or clothes.

The essences are usually applied externally and used commonly in massage. This is thought to allow the essence to travel through the skin to the blood and the body fluids. This permits a slow, gradual absorption in the body. Aromatherapy includes massaging the essential oils mixed with a carrier oil into the body. This is considered to aid in relieving tension and improving circulation.

Remember that most essential oils should be used externally and should not be applied directly onto open cuts or wounds. Most of these oils are meant to be diluted with some form of a carrier oil if being applied directly onto skin. If you choose to use direct, then always do a test patch first.

Remember IF you are pregnant, nursing, or have a serious illness, consult your physician before using essential oils or any other natural product as to avoid possible allergic reaction or other health risks. These and all natural remedies can be potent if not used properly, and even though reactions are rare, they can occur and further research should be done on an individual basis before.

Essential oils have been around for centuries as early as 1500 B.C. and when simply used can really have a positive effect on your mood, health, and environment. This is a simple and inexpensive way to get a good balance and ownership of your day. Having a stressful day at work or at home? Simply sniff or sprinkle some lavender oil around and watch and feel the results of calm come over you.

Proper dilution of oils is as follows:

Children: .5-1% dilution = 3-6 drops of essential oil per ounce of carrier oil such as Almond oil.

Adults: 2.5% dilution = 15 drops of essential oil per ounce of carrier oil. 3% = 20 drops, 5% =30 drops 10% = 60 drops.

ESSENTIAL OILS AND THEIR USES

Basil Oil	Basil oil helps to clear and expel mucus, reduce fever, improve circulation, relieve menstrual cramps, and stimulate menstrual flow.
Bergamot Oil	Bergamot relaxes muscles and reduces pain. It also helps to fight infection, expel mucus, and calm the nerves, as well as aid indigestion. May encourage new tissue growth. DO NOT expose skin to sun after use.
Cedarwood Oil	Cedarwood oil is used by the respiratory system to help ease coughs and reduce the discomforts of colds and flu. It works as an expectorant to expel mucus and congestion. Cedarwood also works to promote urination; functions as an antiseptic to heal wounds and prevent infection; and heal skin problems
Cinnamon Oil	Cinnamon oil is known for its ability to stimulate and warm the body. It can be mixed with a carrier oil and used in massage to promote warmth. DO NOT use during pregnancy.

Chamomile Oil	Chamomile oil has a refreshing, fruity odor. It is used as a general tonic and is soothing to the body and mind. Chamomile oil is often used to relax and relieve stress. It contains anti-inflammatory properties to reduce swelling. Chamomile helps to heal skin conditions such as psoriasis; or eczema. It helps to prevent infection and speeds healing in wounds. It has also been used to ease pain from headaches, and migraines. Chamomile has been in use since the beginning of time and has many spiritual and religious followings in Europe. Christians dedicated Chamomile to Saint Anne, the Mother of the Blessed Virgin Mary.
Clary Sage Oil	Clary sage oil helps to calm the nervous system and relieve depression. It helps to balance the emotions and is a nervous system tonic. It also helps to relieve muscle spasms. DO NOT consume alcohol or use when pregnant.
Cypress Oil	Cypress oil can calm the nervous system and relieve stress. It also helps with pain and muscle aches.
Eucalyptus Oil	Eucalyptus oil is often used with problems associated with colds, allergies, coughs, flu, sinusitis, sore throats and tonsillitis. It is used for sinus complaints and is effective in relieving congestion and a stuffy nose. It is also considered beneficial in helping alleviate the pain of a sore throat. Eucalyptus oil also helps to fight infections, whether viral or bacterial.
Fennel Oil	Fennel oil helps to rid the body of toxins. It is also used to help control the appetite to aid with weight loss. It is used for some female complaints such as irregular menstrual cycle, PMS, fluid retention, and menopausal symptoms.

Frankincense	Frankincense is probably one of the most recognized essential oils and is upheld in Christianity as a "Holy Ointment" it is believed that Egyptians first used frankincense as early as 1500 B.C. and then in the Bible, in Exodus, Moses was instructed by God to use frankincense to make holy incense as he led the Jews out of Egypt. Then again the Three Kings brought Frankincense as one of the gifts to the newborn Jesus.
Geranium Oil	Geranium oil helps with problems such as diarrhea, gallstones, and urinary tract infections. DO NOT use during pregnancy.
Ginger Oil	Ginger oil is commonly used for gastrointestinal disorders. It also helps to increase immunity and protect the body from illness. It stimulates circulation and helps to relieve pain.
Jasmine Oil	Jasmine oil is used to relieve coughs and problems of the female organs. It can be massaged into the lower back to ease the pain from menstrual cramps and induce menstrual flow. Jasmine oil is often recommended to soothe the discomforts of menopause. It has also been used to help ease the pain of childbirth. Jasmine vines and flowers are popular in Florida and smell beautiful in the yard. DO NOT use Jasmine while pregnant, until labor begins.
Juniper Oil	Juniper oil helps to reduce pain and muscle aches. It increases urination and can stimulate menstrual flow. It can fight infection and water retention. DO NOT use during pregnancy.

Lavender Oil	English lavender is considered to be the best type to use when extracting the essential oil. It is used to promote a restful sleep. Lavender oil is a versatile oil used for many conditions. It can be used for digestive problems, respiratory disorders, pain and muscle aches, skin disorders, and wounds. It should be used only in small quantities because of its strong aroma. This calming oil is very popular. Lavender has been used by several ancient religions and is believed to "cleanse."
Lemon Oil	Lemon oil is used for respiratory disorders such as bronchitis, coughs, sore throats, flu and cold symptoms. It contains anti-bacterial properties. It aids in digestion and strengthens the immune system.
Myrrh Oil	Myrrh has been used for thousands of years. It is a sacred oil to boost the immune system, fight infection and heal when an illness is present. It helps with digestion and stimulates the appetite. Some aroma therapists recommend myrrh for respiratory complaints, fungal infections, healing wounds, menstrual complaints, and skin disorders.
Orange Oil	Orange oil helps in relaxing the body. It is used for respiratory problems such as bronchitis, colds and flu. It increases immunity to strengthen the entire body. It is also used to aid digestion, nervous disorders, diarrhea, obesity and muscle and joint aches.
Peppermint Oil	Peppermint is used in cases of fever and headache, and to increase energy levels. It stimulates the nervous system to increase energy and reduce fatigue. It helps with digestion and nausea. It relaxes muscle tension, relieves headaches and migraines, and helps with some skin conditions. DO NOT use during pregnancy.

Rose Oil	A very expensive essential oil. It takes approximately one hundred pounds of petals to extract ½ ounce of oil. This oil is used for digestion, coughs, wound healing, congestion, female hormone balance, skin conditions, headaches, and inflammation. DO NOT use during pregnancy.
Rosemary Oil	Taken from the flowering tops of the plant. It is used for digestion, arthritis, coughs, depression, scalp problems, relaxation, headaches, muscle pain, cardiovascular disorders, respiratory conditions, memory aid, and circulation. Rosemary was considered a sacred plant by the Romans. Christians of the early days believed the rosemary flowers were once white but then turned blue when the Blessed Mother hung her cloak on the rosemary bush on her way to Bethlehem. Rosemary's medieval benefits date back into the 1370's and is believed by some to ward off "evil spirits". NOT to be used during the first four months of pregnancy.
Rosewood Oil	Rosewood oil helps to calm the nervous system. It helps to ease depression, anxiety and stress. It fights infection, increases immunity, relieves pain, and can stimulate sexual desire.
Sandalwood	Sandalwood has been labeled "Oil of Divinity" or "Endless Life" and has been in use since before Christ walked the earth. This oil is believed to give energy and mind strength. Some ancient religions believe sandalwood will purify the body and soul.
Spearmint Oil	Spearmint oil is generally recommended for use with stomach problems. It can aid digestion and help relieve nausea.

Tea Tree Oil	Tea tree oil is well known for its antiseptic properties. It is known to kill infection, whether viral, bacterial or fungal in nature. It is used to treat acne, burns, cuts, dandruff, respiratory ailments, coughs, urinary tract infections, candida, and eczema. This oil comes also in toothpaste, shampoo and mouthwash.
Thyme Oil	Thyme helps to increase immunity and prevent infections. Used mostly for respiratory conditions such as asthma, bronchitis, tonsillitis, coughs, colds, sinusitis, and sore throats. Thyme helps to heal mouth problems such as sore gums and throat infections. It can help increase energy and reduce fatigue. DO NOT use in baths or on skin since this oil can sting.

Healthy Hint: Mandarin Oil is great for calming children and can be combined with lavender oil in a diffuser and the steam will carry into the room creating a calming atmosphere.

Healthy Hint: Patchouli Oil has antidepressant properties as well as anti-inflammatory properties.

Healthy Hint: Just for men, if you need that man cave masculine smell to mark your territory, try a blend of 2 Cypress drops, 2 Wintergreen drops and 2 White Fir drops in a diffuser. It will give a woods like smell.

Healthy Hint: If you're having a low energy day and need a pick me up, try 2 -3 drops of Orange Oil mixed with 2-3 drops of Peppermint Oil. You can use in a diffuser or mix in a carrier oil and dab on.

CHAPTER FIFTEEN
BLOOD TYPES AND PROPER EATING HABITS FOR THEM

EATING RIGHT FOR YOUR BLOOD TYPE

You may have heard a lot about this latest research that seems to indicate that there is a link with blood types and diet. Several of my customers that have followed this type of diet have gotten quite good results.

I neither denounce nor endorse this style of diet, I believe that if you try it and if you feel better, then great it could be right for you. I also do believe that some persons have food allergies to certain foods such as wheat, corn, yeast, gluten and dairy to mention the most common, and by just eliminating these few without totally ignoring any one particular food group may benefit you just as much as following the whole program word for word.

It is my opinion that some of the results these people are getting and the healthier feeling they have can be directly related to controlling unhealthy eating habits and highly allergic foods intake. And I speak as one that knows what food allergies can do to one's health since I myself suffered for several years with food allergies and was on weekly shots for ten years until I changed my eating habits and got on the proper diet, supplements and exercise program.

Find below a brief summary of what the "eat right for your blood type" is all about. Some of the findings are quite interesting, including some, which indicate overcoming disease; effects on aging, stress, energy and many emotional imbalances such as attention deficit disorder and depression can all be improved through this way of eating. It may be something that you wish to experiment with and see how it may work for you.

If you wish to study this subject more in-depth then I suggest you get a copy of Live Right For Your Type, by Dr. Peter J. D'Adamo and Catherine Whitney, out on the market for more details on the blood types and also how to determine your secretor status which could vary your food choices within your very own home, between your blood type and the foods you eat.

BLOOD TYPES

Blood Type "O"

1. This blood type would follow a mostly animal protein diet consisting of lean quality meat several times per week, which has been shown to increase strength, energy and metabolism.

2. Eat cold-water fish, high in rich oils, which improves inflammations, thyroid, metabolism, brain function and much more.

3. Your diet would consist of little or no dairy products since Type O's tend to have a problem with digestion of dairy.

4. Wheat and wheat-based products should be eliminated from your diet. (Ezekiel bread can be used in place of your regular white bread, which does contain wheat.)

5. Try not to consume too many dishes that have beans in them and eat a lot of fruits and vegetables. However avoid high acid foods like oranges.

6. Limit your intake of caffeine and consume pumpkin seeds and walnuts as health snacks.

7. Type "O's" need to be on a regular exercise program, which is crucial for them to stay in-balance emotionally.

Blood Type "A"

1. This blood type would follow a diet consisting mostly of a vegetarian style and would have to avoid excessive red meat intake since it can be hard for Type "A's" to digest and can cause problems with their metabolism.

2. The consumption of poultry such as chicken and turkey would have to be limited to about three times per week and much of the protein intake would be derived from soy products and fresh fish.

3. Cultured dairy products in modest amounts may be included such as yogurt but try to avoid mucous-causing products like fresh milk.

4. Eat plenty of beans and don't indulge in too many wheat-derived foods and avoid

wheat if you can. Consume high amounts of nuts and seeds.

5. Large amounts of fruits and vegetables can be beneficial especially Vitamin "A" rich foods such as carrots, spinach and broccoli.

6. It is important for Type "A"s" to get plenty of sleep and not stay up late. It is also just as important for them to get moving early in the morning. Try not to skip meals but have smaller, more frequent meals throughout the day with more protein early on and less as the day near's end. Some form of cardiovascular exercise is suggested for thirty minutes three times per week such as walking to help calm nerves and aid in digestion.

Blood Type "B"
1. This blood type would follow a varied diet which would include small frequent portions of quality lean meat and richly oiled cold water fish, both of these will help to maintain strength, energy and proper metabolism.

2. Type "B"s" are blessed with a flexible digestive system that will digest carbohydrates and/or animal proteins. Unlike Type "O's" that have high stomach acid and the A's that have low stomach acid.

3. Type "B's" are prone to bacterial infections and safe food preparations are very important. I would suggest adding acidophilus with F.O.S. to your daily supplement intake.

4. Type "B's" also are at risk for memory loss and Alzheimer's later in life so keeping mental activity high is important for mind stimulation.

5. This blood type should avoid chicken, which can easily be replaced with turkey. Additional foods to avoid include corn, buckwheat, lentils, peanuts, tomatoes, and excessive sugar. Type "B's" tend to do well with dairy unlike Type O and Type A. Type B also find eggs a beneficial part of their diets as they do onions and a wide variety of fruits and vegetables.

6. Type "B's" do well with meditation and visualization more so than any other blood type and can use these measures for stress reduction and contributions to their local communities in various ways. Plenty of rest is important as is not skipping meals.

Blood Type "AB"

1. This blood type will have a mixed dietary routine and some of the rules from blood Type A and blood Type B will also apply here with a few additional restrictions.

2. Blood type AB is best when they avoid caffeine and alcohol, especially when in high stress situations. They also should not skip meals.

3. ABs should never skip breakfast and will find it will help balance their metabolic rate and stress levels.

4. This blood type also is known to have low stomach acid, which can cause digestive problems.

5. Type ABs should limit their red meat intake and avoid chicken. A diet high in soy products and most fresh fish would be beneficial.

6. A diet rich in carrots, spinach and broccoli would be best, along with eggs.

7. Foods that should be avoided are chicken, corn, buckwheat, kidney and lima beans. Dairy products can be used with discretion.

8. Blood Type AB's do well with goal planning and gradual changes without over-crowding their agendas. Rest, exercise and group activity is considered beneficial with AB's.

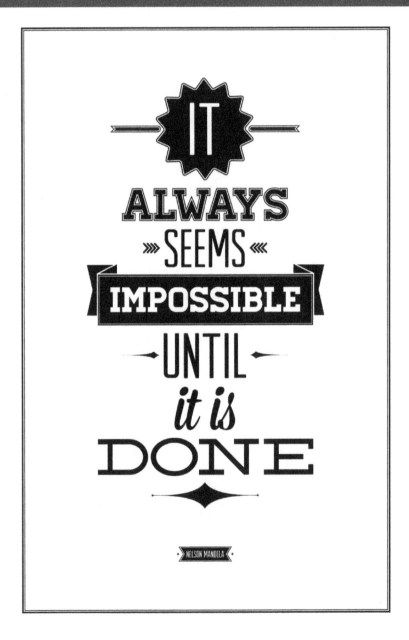

CHAPTER SIXTEEN
OVERLOAD SYNDROME

How to Find Yourself in Today's World

Take a moment and pretend that after tomorrow you won't be around to do any of the things that you normally run around doing and start to make a list of how you think you could delegate all these things to get them done. After all, one day we really won't be here and the world made it through before us and it will make it through after us. We like to think we can't be replaced but the truth of the matter is that everyone can be replaced to some degree. I remember when my aunt became ill and could not return to work, she would run the whole office by herself, going crazy, and then she was stricken with a tumor. Well, when her employer found that she would not be able to return, they ended up replacing her with three people in the office to do all she did. Why didn't she ask for help? The more she did, the more they let her do; and then she ended up sick, replaced and missing a lot of her life and her dreams. Possibly even forgetting what they were.

My point here is that we should communicate our needs. The people that know the job best are the people that are actually doing it, and a lot of times they know better ways of doing things if their voices can be heard. Realize that some changes can be made to accommodate taking care of yourself and your loved ones better and for making time for your health. Here are some ideas for you to consider and they can be implemented over a period of time:

1. Let's say that you and your spouse want to get in a workout three days per week but there seems to be no time. Well, one of you can work out on Tuesday/Thursday/Saturday and the other could workout Monday/Wednesday/Friday, either in the early A.M. while the other one of you readies the kids for school, or in the P.M., as the other gets the kids' dinner and homework done. You could even do this on the same day but in a split shift. One of you gets A.M. duty and the other P.M. duty.

2.   Take out an ad in your children's school newspaper or at your church or local YMCA and see if there is another parent in the same crunch as you that would be willing to work with you in sharing the responsibility of getting the kids either to or from school and homework started. This could work out great and remember we're only talking three hours per week here. You may even try setting up some type of group exercise class within your local neighborhood, put some flyers and signs out and see what interests it draws.

3.   See if your employer is interested in implementing a Flex-Time schedule in which on certain days you can start earlier and leave earlier and possibly not take your lunch that day (still eat but at your desk while working) this could work well for several of you and will help you to avoid rush hour traffic, which will give you more time right there.

4.   Try moving closer to work, closer to a fitness facility. The YMCA offers family passes that can occupy your children with activities while you get your workout in, and you can make it a special family time activity. Remember it doesn't have to be a long workout. Rather, focus on the consistency of making it a set day and time and sticking to it.

5.   Divide the chores up around the house so everyone does a little and this way it will all get done throughout the week and not all hit you at once on your day off. This will free your time up. In fact, it's great to clean the house in sections. Monday and Tuesday maybe the bedrooms, Wednesday, the family room and so on.

6.   Prepare your families' meals and lunches in advance and have everything ready in containers for each day of the week. As an example you can cook up several chicken breasts in advance on Sunday and then refrigerate and re-heat well. Also other foods that do well prepared in advance are meat loaf, tuna and chicken salads, tossed salads (without the dressing until ready to eat), brown rice, hard boiled eggs, cut vegetables and so on.

7. Have everyone's clothes ready to go in advance, pressed, organized, and even labeled for the day of the week. Make your children a part of the process; have them do some of the preparations.

8. Cut out television programs that aren't your favorite and watch only the things you really want to and tape the rest to watch on another day when you may have free time or just disregard altogether. Limit online computer time.

9. Maybe there's even an inexpensive housekeeper and lawn maintenance company that you can find to help you out if it's affordable to you. This seems to free up a few hours per week. You may also be able to work out some type of trade for this service – maybe there's a service you can do that they need.

10. Get to bed earlier and rise earlier and you can get your workout in at home first thing in the morning and be done while everyone else is just getting up.

11. Take time to pray each morning and every night. How can the day possibly go right if you haven't prayed about it? And be confident, after that prayer that you <u>will</u> have a great day.

12. Make the time for church. We seem to make the time for everything else, yet when it comes down to the final day of the final hour, there is only you and God. So try not to put things before him. After all, we're only asking for one hour each Sunday.

13. For those of you that say you can't afford some of the extras yet you have a cell phone and possibly some bad habits like smoking, drinking, playing lottery tickets, renting movies, etc. Well, I can assure you that if you give some of those things up you could afford some of the ideas I've mentioned. Even taking all your credit cards and putting them into a refinance on your mortgage, or even a small second mortage would allow you to get rid of that interest that usually runs 18% to 28% and you cut it to approximately 5-9% which would save you enough to afford other

healthier benefits for your lifestyle. And you'd even be able to write the mortgage interest off at the end of the year, unlike credit card interest. This way you save even more money.

14. Take the time to enjoy your life now and your family now. Develop that special relationship with them and with God. There is no amount of money that is worth losing touch with your loved one, God and yourself. When it comes to the last minute of your breath, you won't care much about what paperwork is on your desk at the office. You will care, however, about having your loved ones at your side.

15. It's amazing that some of the poorest people in the world have some of the greatest relationships with God and their families. Why you may ask? Well, it's because their minds and lives aren't so very cluttered with lots of bills, hectic work schedules and living outside their means. They do not care about the "material-world" and this allows them to take the time to find the true meaning of life. Now take time to re-evaluate your individual situations and make time for each other, yourself and God.

Remember …

Where there's a will —

There's a way…

Take the time for you today.

Workout! Why? Because you're worth it!

CHAPTER SEVENTEEN
TAKING OWNERSHIP OF YOUR CHILDREN'S HEALTH

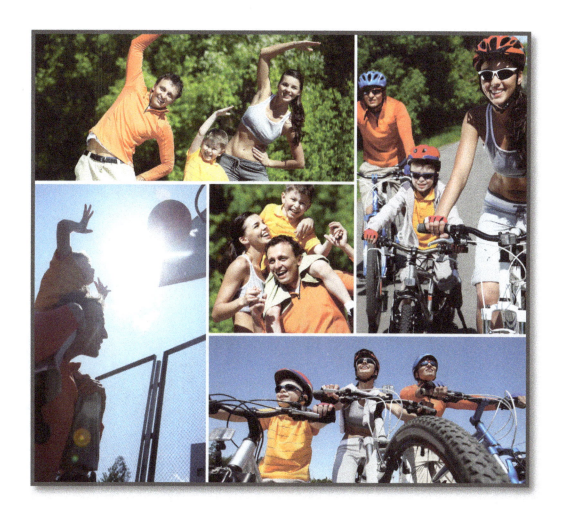

CHAPTER SEVENTEEN
TAKING OWNERSHIP OF YOUR CHILDREN'S HEALTH

"Family Household Fitness"

Build your children up

to reach for their dreams.

Yet keep them grounded in

a foundation of

love, respect, faith, hope

and forgiveness.

Teach them, listen to them,

Hear them and be with them.

Guide them and lead them.

Be an example,

be <u>their</u> example,

<u>be a parent</u>.

Children are unique, children are special. Some have brown hair with matching brown eyes. Others have silky blond hair with bright blue eyes. But they all, no matter what color hair, or what color skin, they all have so much in common. They ALL are the FUTURE.

Each one of them will play a role "somewhere out there" in this world. Some will be doctors, others lawyers. Some will be mayors, others will develop new technologies to save lives. Some will go on to be preachers, others hard laborers, and some even a President of this great nation.

Yes, children are so very alike. They all want LOVE, children need to know they are loved and to be reminded of it on a daily basis. Children need HOPE. They need to know that they can have the opportunity at hand to do great things with their lives. Children need FAITH, they need to know God is there for them through all the ups and downs life has to offer and that their good deeds will be rewarded and that they are promised everlasting life through the death and resurrection of Christ Jesus. CHILDREN will also undoubtedly need FORGIVENESS as all kids do for their early childhood silly mistakes. They will always need to learn and know forgiveness all through their lives so as to let their love shine through and so they too may be forgiven by God for their sins.

Children need to be taught RESPECT, for their parents, teachers, elders, family and friends. It amazes me how kids have a "sixth sense." They are very aware of what is going on around them; they evaluate their parents on a daily basis and are very observant. This is why parents, too, need to be on **THEIR** best behavior. If a parent talks badly of someone, then the child thinks it's okay to do so too. It's really something how we want to raise our kids to be good. Yet on so many occasions we teach them how to be bad and then wonder what went wrong. Think about it. Kids hear their parents talk about trying to avoid paying taxes. They learn early on if it's cheating to the government it's "okay," "because everyone does it." Then they see their parents speeding and not obeying the laws and that's considered "okay," "because everyone does it." Kids learn how to cheat, steal, lie, slander and disrespect everything from their government and leaders to their grandparents and neighbors, to other's faith backgrounds without ever having to leave home. Then we wonder why some children grow up with bad morals and no respect. You're not only raising your child, your teaching them how to raise their children with the values and traditions you are teaching. The next generation, what you do today with your children can have a huge impact for years to come, and this is also true in fitness and nutrition as well, it starts at home.

REMEMBER – YOUR CHILDREN ARE LISTENING!

Children from one end of this earth to the other enjoy a birthday party with balloons and a cake with candles, that special toy for Christmas. They want life's simple pleasures that they will remember for many years to come. Kids want to be kids and enjoy it while they can because it's such a very short part of their lives. Yet in today's society, children are being moved into adulthood very fast and this is where parents can make a difference in their kids' lives.

There is nothing more important than your children. Remember that years from now when a child reaches adulthood and looks back on his or her childhood it will not be the fancy car that their Mom or Dad drove to work every day that they will remember. It is always the more simple things that seem to be the treasures of the childhood memories such as Mom's homemade apple pie, fresh baked cookies for the holidays, the train set Dad helped you put together, the funny looking Christmas tree that you had to make look good and even some discipline too that will be respected later in life when it's better understood (such as getting your butt spanked for talking back}. Your kids will never treasure a memory of you saving for their college tuition as you left home with your briefcase for a 12- hour day and then showed up back at home in a bad mood from work and took it out on them. Telling them how hard you work to give them everything they have doesn't matter to them. Children can't comprehend this and guess what? They don't have to because they're KIDS!

In today's world it seems no one wants to wait for what their parents had later in life. They want it **NOW**. Four kids equal four bedrooms, not two bedrooms with two beds each, like it used to be. Right there a standard of materialism is being introduced to the child at an early age. They already have their own "mini apartment" at ten years old, their "own space" and your parenting starts to become less important to them as you give them more and more independence and they see you less and less. In today's world the children seem to expect it all, or it's time to reorganize a few things until you get a balance that accommodates the household. Just because we can doesn't mean we should when it comes to giving the kids all they want. Teach them to value what they have so they appreciate the things they are given.

We all need heroes in our lives. Take the time and make an effort to be your child's hero. Don't be left behind; now that daycare is considered an essential. Both parents working to make a mortgage payment on a house that is way too expensive. Kids want high priced computer games and are getting them. They have no concept of money. Children are being loaded down with extra homework at an early age with less free time. Parents are expected to rush home from work, do dinner, household duties, shop, clean and help with homework too, and everyone is yelling "Attention Deficit Disorder" A.D.D. for short. How can we start to fix this? Not by covering it up with medication, that's for sure.

ORGANIZATION, PRIORITIZATION and TIME MANAGEMENT will all be a great beginning into "Family Household Fitness."

Remember, in most cases you get out of it what you put into it. Are you your child's hero? There seems to be less and less "Hero types" for our children and even ourselves to look up to now a days. We must all keep some kid in us and still have fun in life and balance the stress. Never go a holiday with putting up decorations and celebrating life, we never know when it will be our last one, never assume you can do it 'next year" because at some point yourself or someone you love might not be here, so celebrate.

When it comes to people to look up to, particularly to blame is the media news and print organizations and even the world of politics. It seems as soon as we have someone to feel good about, then someone else is out there trying to dig something bad up on the person to tear them down. If they would only stick to the issues instead of the personal attacks, it is okay to disagree, that is what this great country is about, our freedom and right to debate our own views.

Children are known for developing their personality traits at a very young age, I believe that even self esteem, self worth, family traditions, values, respect, religion, manners, eating habits and fitness awareness can all be taught at an early age and instilled as a lifestyle. Just as easily as bad habits are picked up, so are good habits. How many times have parents that are raising toddlers that are just beginning to talk, heard them spit out a bad word that shocks the parents. And the parents say "what did you say?" Even at a very young age children take on their parents' habits, both good and bad. So let's try and make all the habits good around the children. And here are some tips. These will help you along the way. Make sure it starts with respect of their own bodies and what impression it gives of themselves, their parents. Make sure they dress respectfully. Children must feel accountable for how they present themselves; it will make a difference in all parts of their lives and yours too.

1. Say a blessing before dinner each and every night. So simple, yet not many families do it on a regular basis. Teach your children to be thankful for each and every meal, every time they are able to come home to a place to live with all the comforts that we take for granted. It also teaches them daily that we are accountable for our daily actions and all these small traditions help you instill respect and a certain level of control, if they listen to you on small things then they are more likely to listen on the bigger issues. And make sure that no cell phones are aloud at the dinner table.

2. Have your children each pick one good thing that they're going to do for someone else that week, free of charge.

3. Let each one of your kids pick an exercise for the whole family to partake in each week, getting them into the habit of a fitness pattern as a way of life. As an example: Julie chose that on this Friday after dinner that the whole family would walk around the block. Then Tommy choses the following week that Saturday the whole family would go into the back yard and do ten jumping jacks and sit ups and a few other things on a small obstacle course you let him put together for all of you. It may not seem like much but it will get them into the frame of mind that exercise is a part of life even if for 15 minutes and, who knows, after a couple months you may all be jogging around the block.

4. Have your kids pick one healthy meal they cook and one healthy dessert to have each week. Call, say Wednesday, your health day and have your kids take turns with

you on preparing something healthy to eat. This way they start to become aware of good quality foods instead of only fried chicken and French fries.

5. Choose a "cheat meal day" for the whole family to have whatever they want that day. This makes it easier to get through the rest of the week eating healthy and save the "cheat" day as a reward. It will help them avoid junk food temptations during the week.

6. All children should be on a good multi-vitamin for children. Stay away from the common grocery store children's vitamins, which tend to be filled with synthetic vitamins, food dyes, chemical sweeteners and junk type fillers. I have found "Nutrastars"-Fruit Blast from Rainbow Light and "Animal on Parade" from Nature's Plus to be of good quality and liked by the children.

7. Teach your children responsibility for money. Sometimes they ask for expensive items because they do not understand that it is very expensive. They have no concept of money, or they think you can write a check or charge it, not realizing that you still have to pay. It is my recommendation that, as your children get older, you let them take part in the family budget. Let them sit down and try to balance the bills with you, make a family chart showing the income you choose to have as a total for the family that month and then list out each of the bills, misc. expenses, etc., and let them see what is left for play and see if they can come up with solutions such as:
    A.   Washing your car instead of taking it to the car wash
    B.   Turning off the lights to save on the electric bill.
    C.   Limiting time on Facebook and cell phone use.

8. See if some of the parents near where you live will have a study group for homework so each night you can each take turns having the kids do their homework at the neighbors on a certain night after school. This will give each of you more time and will be less stressful.

9. Get involved in the school board meetings in your communities and see if there is a

way to cut down on some homework that may not be as important. As we continue to live in an information overload age, some older basics may be needing a phase-out to make room for newer studies that are needed for this new age we live in.

10. Make sure that labels are read on the foods, try to limit sodas and high sugar items from the children's diets. Try not to fry foods when you can bake them. Don't overload the carbohydrates at night, such as pasta, bread and potatoes. Your dinner will be just great with a skinless baked or grilled chicken breast, green salad with low cal dressing, a vegetable and possibly a small portion of brown rice.

11. Introduce them to Christian music; it's come a long way. There are great artists from mellow to rock that will help feed their minds with good messages in a performance that will be fun and exciting.

12. Make sure your children get into the habit of attending church every Sunday. Find a church that offers a variety of programs for yourself and your children. My church offers a "Life Teen" service for young adults that is filled with great music and a great message. It's wonderful to attend and see the youth of today, tomorrow's future, praising and worshiping God hand in hand. It does make a difference.

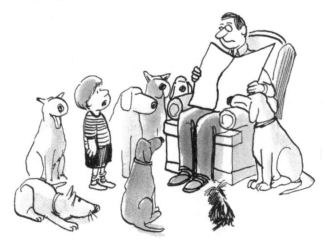

"Dad, the team feels your feeding leadership
is lacking."

CHAPTER EIGHTEEN
FITNESS TERMS TO KNOW

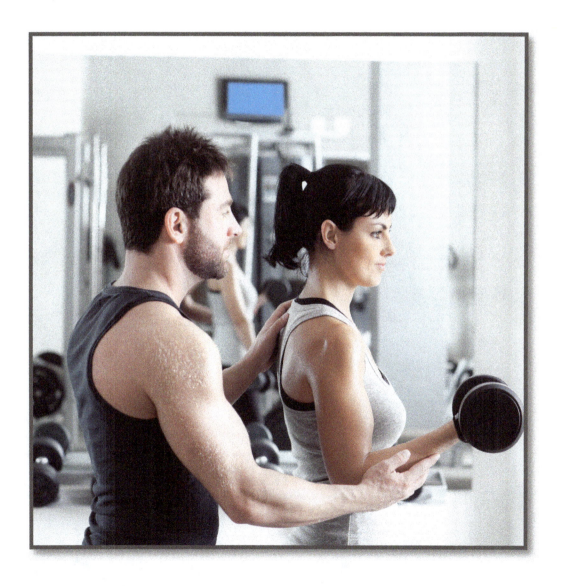

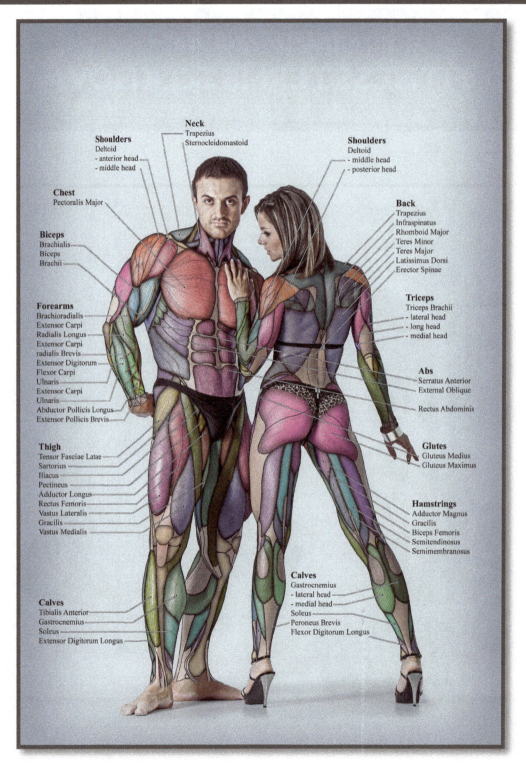

Neck
Trapezius
Sternocleidomastoid

Shoulders
Deltoid
- anterior head
- middle head

Shoulders
Deltoid
- middle head
- posterior head

Chest
Pectoralis Major

Back
Trapezius
Infraspinatus
Rhomboid Major
Teres Minor
Teres Major
Latissimus Dorsi
Erector Spinae

Biceps
Brachialis
Biceps
Brachii

Forearms
Brachioradialis
Extensor Carpi
Radialis Longus
Extensor Carpi
radialis Brevis
Extensor Digitorum
Flexor Carpi
Ulnaris
Extensor Carpi
Ulnaris
Abductor Pollicis Longus
Extensor Pollicis Brevis

Triceps
Triceps Brachii
- lateral head
- long head
- medial head

Abs
Serratus Anterior
External Oblique

Rectus Abdominis

Thigh
Tensor Fasciae Latae
Sartorius
Iliacus
Pectineus
Adductor Longus
Rectus Femoris
Vastus Lateralis
Gracilis
Vastus Medialis

Glutes
Gluteus Medius
Gluteus Maximus

Hamstrings
Adductor Magnus
Gracilis
Biceps Femoris
Semitendinosus
Semimembranosus

Calves
Gastrocnemius
- lateral head
- medial head
Soleus
Peroneus Brevis
Flexor Digitorum Longus

Calves
Tibialis Anterior
Gastrocnemius
Soleus
Extensor Digitorum Longus

Fast-Twitch Fibers

This term simply refers to muscle cells that respond more quickly and are used primarily when you do aerobic activities such as sprinting, etc.

Slow-Twitch Fibers

This refers to muscle cells that contract slowly and that are more resistant to fatigue. These muscle fibers come into play during endurance activities such as long distance running and cycling.

Pump

This term is used a lot by weight lifters and it refers to the muscle being worked swelling with blood and tightening the skin in that particular muscle group making it "pumped up" or larger during and after the workout and this pump usually lasts about two hours after training and it also allows you to know that you were working the targeted muscle group.

Peaking

Any exercise that allows you to achieve maximum isolation on a specific muscle being worked or a body builder preparing for competition that has achieved maximum muscle definition.

Burns

This term is used when you do two or three short partial reps at the end of your regular set. You may hear the term "go for the burn" it basically means that on those extra reps you've added, you have brought extra blood and lactic acid into the muscle, causing a bit of discomfort know as a "burn." This helps to make sure you've maxed out the muscle group, which will contribute to added size and vascularity.

Forced Reps

The reps should be used only after you've completed as many reps as you can achieve on your own. Then your training partner can step in to help you get an extra one or two reps to make sure you've worked out to your maximum capacity for that particular muscle group and it can also be left just for your final set of each exercise.

Visualization

This term can be quite beneficial to you during your training. What this means is to visualize the muscle you're training at looking how you wish it to be. This has been shown to help speed up results. As an example, if you want a defined waistline then visualize and picture those as muscles in your mind. If you want larger biceps visualize your biceps round and bulging. This can also be referred to as the "mind link" and can have a great impact on your success.

Form

This is very important. Proper form is more important than how much weight you're lifting. Perfect form means to involve only the muscles in the exercise description. As an example, on the bicep curl, only lift the weight up using the bicep strength, not by jerking the waist up using your back muscles (and risking injury and usually achieving no muscle pump).

Repetition (also referred to as a Rep)

This means EACH count of an exercise that is being performed. That means every time you've raised the weight and then brought it back to the starting position.

Set

This means a particular grouping of repetitions followed by a rest period. So you may raise the weight eight times then rest; that would be considered one set. Most exercises have three to five sets before moving on to the next movement.

Aerobic Exercise

This term is the prolonged, moderate to intense workouts that use up oxygen at or below the level which a person's cardio respiratory system can replenish the oxygen into the muscles being worked. Now this is the only type of exercise that burns body fat to meet its energy needs. This type of exercise helps to build the lung and heart fitness as well as burning off excess body fat. This majorly helps with one's endurance and energy levels throughout the day.

I strongly recommend getting the aerobic/cardio activity in at least three days per week for thirty minutes, even if you need to start with twenty minutes the first two weeks, from which you will still benefit.

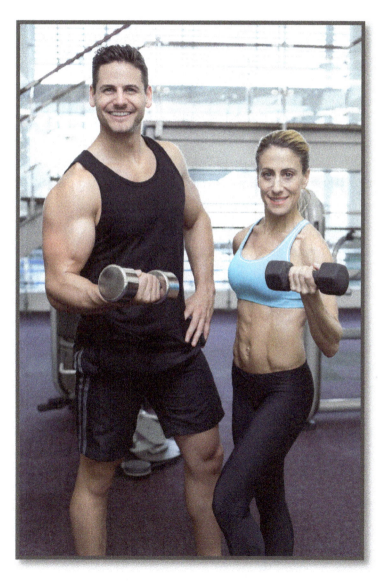

PROPER ETIQUETTE IN THE GYM

1. Dress in a T-shirt and shorts, or gym clothes that have your body covered so you do not sweat all over the equipment and/or make other people feel uncomfortable. If you're making a commitment to workout in a public gym, then have respect for the public by dressing properly or simply workout at home. There will be plenty of time to show off the gym body at the beach or after the gym. Still look good, but make it about the workout and not about a social or fashion show and do not tuck your shirt in, anytime I see this it tells me they already planned on a light workout and come on guys…spandex went out years ago with the Jane Fonda workout, don't do it!

2. DO NOT take your cell phone onto the gym equipment and talk or answer calls while in the middle of your workout. If you must bring your phone, kindly take the call in the lobby, or simply step outside to call them back. Many people talk very loudly on their phones and it really distracts from other people's workouts, and it distracts your workout, too. If something is going on that is so important that you are waiting for a call, perhaps it is best to wait for the call, then do your workout later, when you're more focused. You're not properly working out at the gym when you're talking on the phone, and you distract others from their workouts, too. Again, if you join a public gym, then have respect for the public. Understand that other members might be looking from a distance waiting for the machine you're on, so don't take time socializing or resting too long between sets.

3. Bring a towel to wipe off the equipment if your gym does not provide you with one. Even if you plan on wiping the machines with a paper towel when you're done, this will not work well when the gym is busy since other people might ask to work in with you in between your sets and it will be a problem if the equipment is all sweaty. Remember, everyone else pays for their membership just like you do, so the equipment and machines are for their use too. So again, if you choose to work out in a public place, then show the proper courtesy to others.

4. Wash your hands often or use the sanitizer. Even though the gym cleans the equipment daily, people are touching, sweating, sneezing, and coughing on it and there are germs, so make sure you protect yourself and others by keeping your hands clean.

5. Respect the locker rooms and keep them clean. Flush the toilets and urinals. Wear a towel if you are going to shave, do your hair, or just hang out a bit in the locker room, because no one needs to see all the private stuff that should be private. Again, this is a public place, not your home, so respect the shared space. You might not mind, but others do. No gum-spitting into the urinals, guys, and no gum stuck to the bottom of the machines. Put your garbage in the waste receptacles, and try wiping down the counter if you make a huge mess washing up. Clean out your gym bags regularly so the place doesn't stink. It's amazing this stuff happens when most of the gym members are adults.

6. Try not to yell and throw weights. First of all, the yelling distracts others around you, and the throwing of weights could injure someone, including yourself. It is fine to grunt and groan, but some members take it too far and like to get attention. You're not working out any harder by yelling. The weight does not increase on the bar, it is already on there. Get a spotter for the heavy forced lifts and respect the equipment which often breaks and will be out of use for a week for other members.

7. Do not wear heavy colognes since it stays on the machines when you sweat, then the next person picks up your scent. Many people have allergies to colognes.

8. Remember that the sauna, steam room, jacuzzi and shower do not count as workout time.

CHAPTER NINETEEN
GOAL SETTING

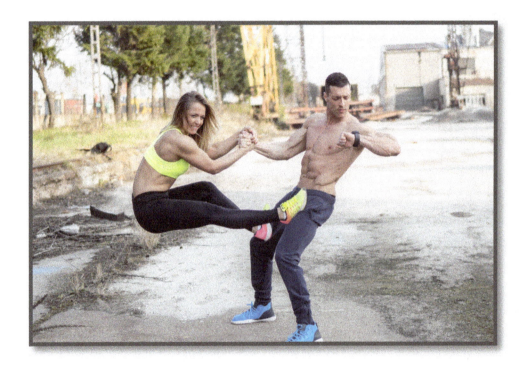

CHAPTER NINETEEN
GOAL SETTING

KEEPING IT SIMPLE = SUCCESS

Keeping it simple equals success in many cases. One of the biggest misconceptions I have witnessed in the nutrition and fitness industry, is that people try going directly from doing no exercise routine, no diet plan and no supplements, to jumping right in and going overboard into everything at once and at maximum levels. What happens shortly there after when they are into this four to six weeks or so, is that they get stressed with the work load, they start to miss workouts and go off their diet plans. Before they know it, they are right back to where they started again. This is called roller coaster dieting and exercise, up and down over and over again. Sound familiar? I'm sure you know someone that does this, or maybe you do it yourself.

Remember, more is not always better, especially in a fitness and diet routine for the average person that has a job and family to deal with too. There are no quick fixes when it comes to getting in true shape. You must own your body and make a true lifestyle change and not a quick fix. Fitness must become a way of life, not just something you borrow to make yourself feel better for trying. Then you complain that nothing works for you. Own up to what you have to do to make a better you and do it today!

Just do it! It is better to take on a realistic fitness program and diet plan that you are more likely to stay with and can be consistent with. It may take a bit longer to achieve your results, but the results will last and your life with change because you changed.

Being consistent in your program is the key, being balanced. If you have a longer work day and more family obligations on Wednesday's, then don't put your workout on that day. If you do, you're just setting yourself up to fail. Be realistic, know your schedule. Plan your week out in advance on a chart and stay organized. You must know where you're going each week if you expect to get there; otherwise, you're just driving your fitness and nutrition program in circles and never getting out of the car. It's time to park the car, walk your butt into the gym or fitness class and make it happen. If it starts with Zumba or Jazzercise classes two or three times a week, that's fine, just get yourself into a routine and train yourself to stay with a program and then branch out to a bigger program when you've accomplished the basics. Let this fitness routine, no matter how small or large, become a part of who you are. OWN IT!

It is always better to do a program two or three days a week and stay with it for life, than it is to do a heavy program five to six days a week and stay with it for a month. Building a program set around your life that is realistic and truly for you is the first great step to accomplishing your long term goals. Every success story has a beginning.

So now let's look at this. As an example, if you don't like or eat fish then don't put it in your daily diet plan because your brain will associate it with pain and you will find a reason not to eat it. Just add some flaxseed oil and fish oil pills to your daily vitamin intake so you still get those good healthy oils in your diet. Replace it with a grilled chicken breast. If you don't like gyms, then you must go at an off time when less people are there, or workout at home. If you don't like a gym and try going between 4:00pm – 7:00pm when it is the busiest, then you will miss workouts. Again be realistic about what you are doing and when, and where you're doing it. Thirty minutes on a lifecycle in front of your television is better than walking up to the gym at 5:00pm and walking away because if you're a woman you feel fat when the girls are running around in short-shorts or if you're a guy, guys are wearing tank tops and your gut is hanging out and then that makes you self-conscious to the point that you will think you need to get in better shape before you go to the gym. That's crazy, because that is why you need the gym in the first place. Just get to the root of what is holding you back and then find what you can do to accomodate it. People find off the wall excuses, but it is all true. On the inside we really do want to look our best and we really do care what other's think about us. So simply put, start with something simple and comfortable and ease your way into a true routine and lifestyle change. Start to train your brain and body that this is something you do now, you workout. Trust me, you're going to feel so much better physically and mentally that you are doing something for your health and for you. We all need "our time," just a little space for ourselves, so make sure you own that little space for yourself starting today.

Realistic Goals

As you continue to get into the best shape of your life, remember this very important part. Concentrate on what you can do, and what you can be. If you're always worrying that you'll never be a size five because of your structure, then just work on being the best size eight there is. If you men simply can't achieve a 30-inch waist, then have a great looking, well toned 32 or 33-inch waist. If you're always worrying about what others can accomplish above and beyond what you can, then in most cases this will only cause non-productive frustration it will only hold you back and not advance you onto your future achievements. Set realistic goals.

Goal setting is best accomplished when you first come up with exactly what it is that you want to do. Maybe lose fifty pounds or lose two inches on your waist. It could also be about gaining two more inches of muscle on your chest and arms, and so on. So first get a notebook, or use the charts I've provided, and let's get busy on goal setting.

Write down what you are setting out to accomplish long term by, let's say, this time next year. Then we go into dividing this up into 12 week cycles. It will better serve you to have three short term goals, each four weeks long. This will equal the one large goal when it is completed. Plus, this will help keep you motivated seeing progress and mini-goals achieved every four weeks.

Next find a picture or two of what you would realistically like to look like. Cut it out of a magazine. Tape one on your refrigerator and another someplace where you frequently are. Then decide on a starting day. Take all of your measurements and weight and write them on the chart I've provided.

FITNESS GOALS

List four separate goals that would be considered "short-term goals" that will eventually equal your "long-term goals." Example: Long-term goals may be to lose six inches off your waist, so divide this up into three separate short-term goals which will keep you motivated and focused on your end result. This would have your goal at losing two inches off your waist every four weeks. Twelve weeks is enough time to make a true body transformation.

Goal #1 (End of first four-week cycle)

Goal #2 (End of second four-week cycle)

Goal #3 (End of third four-week cycle)

Now, you may take this into a second phase if need be and select a new set of goals to achieve your next level.

Remember, you have to know where you're going before you can get there!

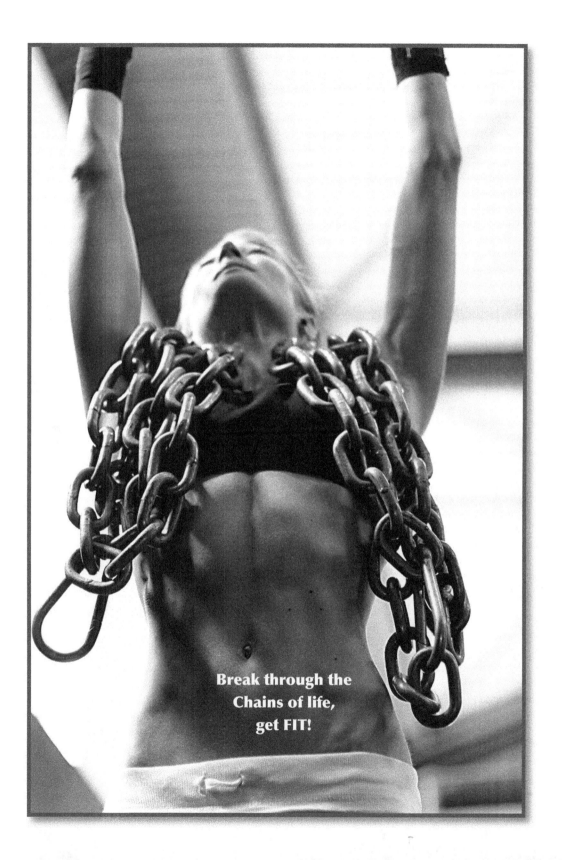

Break through the
Chains of life,
get FIT!

TAKE YOUR "BEFORE" PICTURES AND MEASUREMENTS

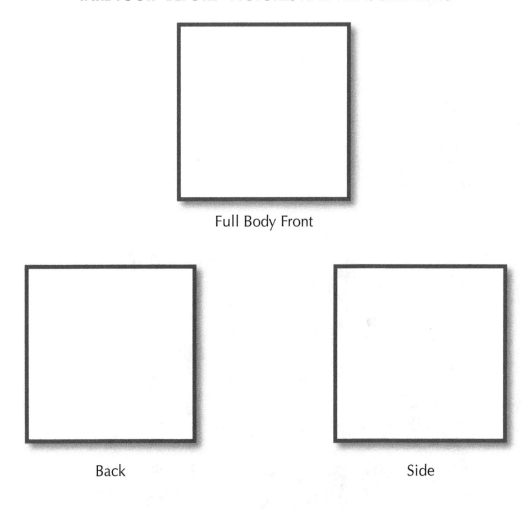

Full Body Front

Back   Side

Height: Arms:

Weight: Body Fat %:

Chest: Shirt/Blouse Size:

Waist: Dress Size:

Thigh: Slacks/Pants Size:

Hips:

TAKE YOUR "AFTER" PICTURES AND MEASUREMENTS

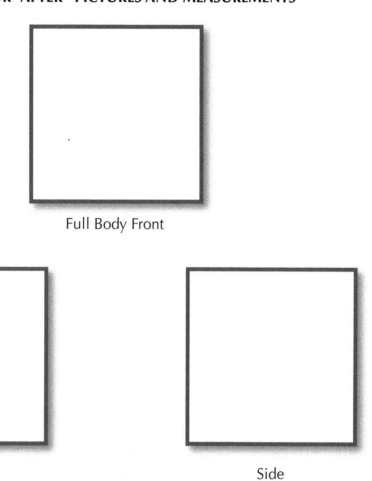

Full Body Front

Back   Side

Height: Arms:

Weight: Body Fat %:

Chest: Shirt/Blouse Size:

Waist: Dress Size:

Thigh: Slacks/Pants Size:

Hips:

PLACE A REALISTIC PICTURE HERE OF SOMEONE YOU WANT YOUR BODY TO LOOK LIKE AS YOUR GOAL AND MOTIVATION.

If you want
something
you've never had,
you must be willing
to do
SOMETHING
you've never
DONE!

CHAPTER TWENTY
BUILDING YOUR WORKOUT ROUTINE

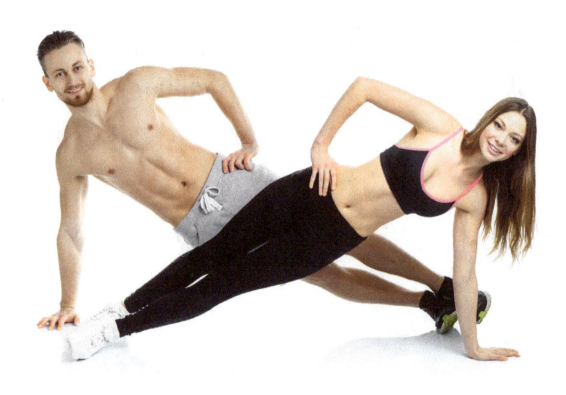

CHAPTER TWENTY
BUILDING YOUR WORKOUT ROUTINE

MEN'S & WOMEN'S ROUTINES

These programs are to be done 2-3 days per week. For weight gain, use heavier weight and the lower rep range. For weight/fat loss and leaner muscle and more cuts, use lighter weight and higher rep range. As soon as your last rep gets too easy, then you need to add weight or increase reps depending on what you want to achieve. If you do not have access to machines, then you may substitute with free weight exercise and vice versa.

Remember to add three 30-40 minutes sessions of cardio where your time allows on separate days or the same day if possible. Doing cardio on an empty stomach first thing in the morning or at least 2 hours after food will allow your body to burn stored fat as an energy source, which will allow you to lose body fat faster. Make sure you get a quality protein shake with amino acids after your workout and cardio day. This will allow you to recover faster and not burn muscle, but repair and recover muscle tissue leading to your physique goals.

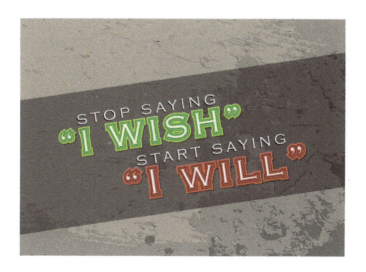

KEEPING IT SIMPLE, JUST BEGINNER BASICS
MEN'S 3-DAY PER WEEK WORKOUT PLAN

EXERCISES Warm up 10 min.	MON. Life Cycle	WED. Treadmill	FRI. Elliptical
	SETS/REPS	SETS/REPS	SETS/REPS
CHEST			
Barbell Flat Bench Press	2-3 8-15	========	========
Dumbbell Incline Press	========	2-3 8-15	========
Dumbbell Flyes	========	========	2-3 8-15
SHOULDERS			
Barbell Upright Row	2-3 8-15	========	========
Barbell Press Behind Neck	========	2-3 8-15	========
Dumbbell Side Laterals	========	========	2-3 8-15
ARMS			
Dumbbell Alternate Bicep Curls	2-3 8-15	========	========
Preacher Curls - Machine	========	2-3 8-15	========
Concentration Curls - Dumbbell	========	========	2-3 8-15
BACK			
Lat Pulldown - Machine	2-3 8-15	========	2-3 8-15
One Arm Dumbbell Row	========	2-3 8-15	========
TRICEP			
Tricep Pushdown	2-3 8-15	========	2-3 8-15
Seated Tricep Extension	========	2-3 8-15	========
LEGS			
Barbell Squat	2-3 8-15	========	========
Machine Leg Press	========	2-3 8-15	========
Machine Leg Extension	========	========	2-3 8-15
Machine Leg Curl	========	========	2-3 8-15
CALVES			
Machine Calf Raises	2-3 8-15	========	2-3 8-15
Toe Presses	========	2-3 8-15	========
ABS			
Floor Crunches	2-3 20-25	========	2-3 20-25
Side Twists	2-3 20-25	========	========
Leg Raises	========	2-3 20-25	========
Machine Seated Ab Crunch	========	2-3 20-25	========
Side Bends	========	========	2-3 20-25

KEEPING IT SIMPLE, JUST THE BIGINNER BASICS
WOMEN'S 3-DAY PER WEEK WORKOUT PLAN

EXERCISES	MON.	WED.	FRI.
Warm up 10 min.	Life Cycle	Treadmill	Elliptical
	SETS/REPS	SETS/REPS	SETS/REPS
CHEST			
Dumbbell Flat Bench Press	2-3 8-15	========	========
Dumbbell Incline Press	========	2-3 8-15	========
Dumbbell Flyes	========	========	2-3 8-15
SHOULDERS			
Seated Dumbbell Overhead Press	2-3 8-15	========	========
Dumbbell Side Laterals	========	2-3 8-15	========
Dumbbell Front Raise	========	========	2-3 8-15
ARMS			
Dumbbell Alternate Bicep Curl	2-3 8-15	========	2-3 8-15
Dumbbell Concentration Curl	========	2-3 8-15	========
BACK			
Single Dumbbell Row or	2-3 8-15	========	2-3 8-15
Lat pulldown	========	2-3 8-15	========
TRICEP			
Tricep Pushdown	2-3 8-15	========	2-3 8-15
Seated Dumbbell Kickback	========	2-3 8-15	========
LEGS			
Dumbbell Squat	2-3 8-15	========	========
Dumbbell Lunges or Leg Curl	========	2-3 8-15	========
Leg Extension	========	========	2-3 8-15
Calf Raises	========	2-3 8-15	========
ABS			
Floor Crunches	2-3 20-25	========	2-3 20-25
Side Twists	2-3 20-25	========	========
Side Bends	========	2-3 20-25	========
Leg Raises	========	2-3 20-25	========
Seated Ab Crunch - Machine	========	========	2-3 20-25

If Tuesday, Thursday, and Saturday work better, for both men and women, then use those days and always do 30 minutes of cardio on an empty stomach on three mornings of your off days from training.

The following programs are for use after you have become more advanced in your training and have completed at least 8-12 weeks of your basic program for beginners. You can choose to move on to the next level when you feel that you are no longer challenged by the basic beginner program, or instead you may choose to just exchange some of the exercises in the beginner basic program with some others I've shown in the book to keep you challenged and to keep the routine fresh, shocking the body, and that will keep new results coming.

The advanced programs offer a three-day-on and two-day-off routine, or a four-day split routine. This will allow you to build your own routine if you choose, and to also pick the exercises that will be used for each body part as you become more advanced in your training. This will allow you to specialize each muscle group on your training days; you will be doing more sets than you do with the full body training simply because you will have more time to specialize the training day to fit specific muscle groups. This will truly bring you up to a new fitness level when you get to this advanced form of training. Some of you may choose to use a combination of both or even go back and forth between the different methods of training routines every 12 weeks.

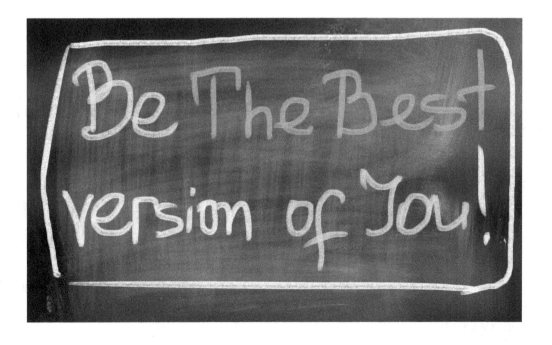

EXAMPLES OF THE THREE-ON / TWO-OFF SPLIT

Alternative 1

Day 1	Day 2	Day 3	Day 4-5
Chest	Legs	Shoulders	Rest
Back	Calves	Arms	
Abdominals	Abdominals	Calves	

Alternative 2

Day 1	Day 2	Day 3	Day 4-5
Chest	Back	Legs	Rest
Shoulders	Biceps	Calves	
Triceps	Abdominals	Abdominals	

EXAMPLES OF THE FOUR-DAY SPLIT

Alternative 1

Monday / Thursday	Tuesday / Friday
Abdominals	Abdominals
Chest	Legs
Deltoids	Arms
Back	Calves

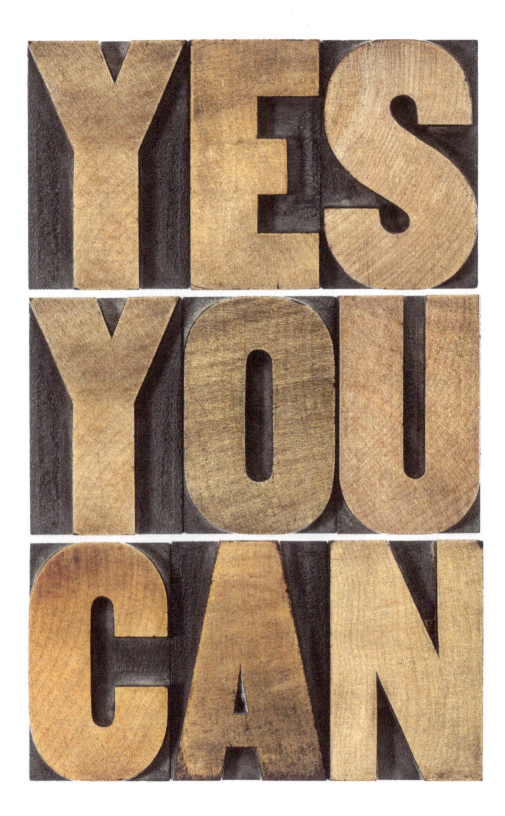

Alternative 2	
Monday / Thursday	**Tuesday / Friday**
Abdominals	Abdominals
Chest	Legs
Shoulders	Back
Arms	Calves

Alternative 3	
Monday / Thursday	**Tuesday / Friday**
Abdominals	Abdominals
Legs	Back
Chest	Deltoids

Endomorph

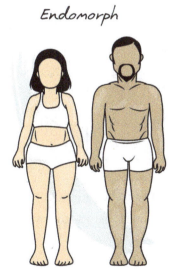

Mesomorph

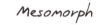
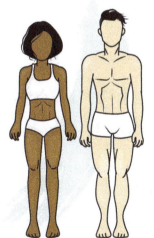

Ectomorph

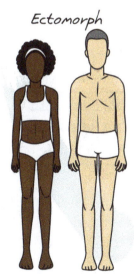

Slower Metabolism   Easy Gain and Loses   Hard Gainer

SAMPLE ROUTINE

Monday and Thursday
SHOULDERS * CHEST * TRICEPS * ABDOMINALS

EXERCISE	BEGINNER		INTERMEDIATE	
	Sets	Reps	Sets	Reps
SHOULDER				
Dumbbell Press or/	1 - 2	8 - 15	3 - 4	8 - 15
Lateral Raises	1 - 2	8 - 15	3 - 4	8 - 15
Upright Rows	1 - 2	8 - 15	3 - 4	8 - 15
BACK				
Pull Downs to Front	1 - 2	8 - 15	3 - 4	8 - 15
Dumbbell Rowing	1 - 2	8 - 15	3 - 4	8 - 15
CHEST				
Bench Press or/	1 - 2	8 - 15	3 - 4	8 - 15
Dumbbell Flyes	1 - 2	8 - 15	3 - 4	8 - 15
Incline Press	1 - 2	8 - 15	3 - 4	8 - 15
TRICEPS				
Tricep Pushdown or/	1 - 2	8 - 15	3 - 4	8 - 15
Dumbbell Kickback	1 - 2	8 - 15	3 - 4	8 - 15
ABDOMINALS				
Leg Raises	2 - 3	20	3 - 4	20
Standing Side Bends	2 - 3	20	3 - 4	20

* For weight loss, toning, and lean muscle mass, use lighter weight and higher repetitions.
* For weight gain and building muscle mass, use heavier weight and lower repetitions.

Tuesday and Friday
LEGS * CALVES * BICEPS * FOREARMS * ABDOMINALS

EXERCISE	BEGINNER		INTERMEDIATE	
	Sets	**Reps**	**Sets**	**Reps**
LEGS				
Squats or/	1 - 2	8 - 15	3 - 4	8 - 15
Leg Extension	1 - 2	8 - 15	3 - 4	8 - 15
Leg Curl	1 - 2	8 - 15	3 - 4	8 - 15
CALVES				
Calf Machine Raises	1 - 2	8 - 15	3 - 4	8 - 15
-or-				
Toe Presses on Leg Press Machine	1 - 2	8 - 15	3 - 4	8 - 15
BICEPS				
Alternate Dumbbell Curl or/	1 - 2	8 - 15	3 - 4	8 - 15
Preacher Bench Curl	1 - 2	8 - 15	3 - 4	8 - 15
Concentration Curl	1 - 2	8 - 15	3 - 4	8 - 15
FOREARMS				
Reverse Curl	1 - 2	8 - 15	3 - 4	8 - 15
ABDOMINALS				
Crunches	2 - 3	20	3-4	25
Knee Ins off bench	2 - 3	20	3-4	25
Standing Side Twists	2 - 3	20	3-4	25

* For weight loss, toning, and lean muscle mass, use lighter weight and higher repetitions.

*For weight gain & building mass, use heavier weight/lower reps

EXERCISE LOG

Week of _____

EXERCISES	SETS	REPS	WEIGHT

Comments:

* Make copies of this weekly chart and keep track of your progress.

Create your own workout routine. These exercises can be performed at a gym or if you choose to train at home, you can invest in an adjustable set of dumbbell's and a small weight bench, or see about setting up a full home gym or just use some of the exercises that do not require any equipment.

Remember use the warm-up set of each exercise to familiarize yourself with how to properly conduct the exercise with proper form. This will also allow you to warm the muscle group up since no weight will be used for this set.

Start by picking 2 or 3 exercises per body part and performing 1 warm-up set followed by 3 sets of 8-12 reps.

Lightweight and higher reps work well for weight loss, tone and conditioning.

Moderate to heavy weight and lower reps work well for building up and building mass.

Some people do well combining both these methods. One heavy day and one light day per muscle group.

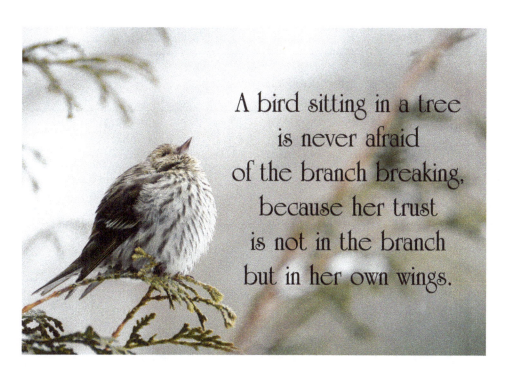

A bird sitting in a tree is never afraid of the branch breaking, because her trust is not in the branch but in her own wings.

BUILD YOUR OWN ROUTINE

Cardio	* Lifecycle * Treadmill * Jogging *Stair Stepper Do 30 minutes of cardio on an empty stomach first thing in the morning on 3 of your non-weight training days and 10 minutes prior to workout.
Stretching	* gently stretch out all muscle groups
Chest	* incline dumbbell press * butter flye * dumbbell flyes * chest pullovers * barbell bench press * dumbbell bench press * decline press * machine chest press
Shoulders	* dumbbell press * seated press behind * side laterals neck * standing barbell press * front dumbbell raise * upright row * dumbbell shrug
Back	* wide-grip pull downs * seated cable row * one-arm dumbbell rows * bent over barbell row
Triceps	* dumbbell extensions * close-grip pushdowns * dumbbell kickbacks
Biceps	* incline dumbbell curls * concentration curl * standing barbell curls * preacher curls * dumbbell curls
Quadriceps	* leg extensions * dumbbell squats * barbell squats * dumbbell squat/dead lift * leg press * hack squat
Hamstrings	* dumbbell lunges * lying leg curls
Calves	* seated calf raises * dumbbell calf raises * standing calf raises * toe raises on leg press machine

Dave's Personal Ab Blaster Routine

Side Twists with broomstick handle

Seated Machine Chair Crunches

Leg Knee Ins off end of bench

Side Bends with broomstick handle

One set of 25 reps of each exercise will be a superset, do not rest in between exercises. Continue and do 4 super sets. This ab routine can be done every morning and you may decide to add an additional evening session if you really want to see some results, 5 days per week.

Dave's Personal Arm Blaster Routine

Preacher Machine Curls 3 sets of 8-10 reps

Alternate Dumbbell Curls 3 sets of 8-10 reps

Concentration DB Curls 3 sets of 8-10 reps

Ticep Pushdowns 3 sets of 8 -10 reps

(Sample of optional drop set to shock the bicep growth)

Start your preacher curl with a comfortable weight to be able to get 8-10 reps, then move the pin and add 10 lbs each set going until you reach your max weight for 10 reps. After your maxed out last set, then immediately drop the weight 10 lbs and lift until failure, then drop another 10 lbs and same thing all the way down to about 40lbs doing each drop set to failure. Your arms will be major pumped and hardly able to move. Do this to shock your biceps about every six weeks it will get some added growth out of it.

On your regular arm day, start with a normal preacher curl with a comfortable weight for 8-10 reps for 3 sets, Superset this with Alternate Dumbbell Curls 8-10 reps and then Superset those with Concentration Dumbbell Curls seated on edge of a bench. Do one set of each for one Superset and repeat 3 times. Contract your bicep at the top of each movement.

Dave's Personal Back Routine

Machine Lat Pull Downs 3 sets of 12 -15 reps

Bent Over Barbell Rows 3 sets of 12 – 15 reps

Seated Machine Pulley Row 3 sets of 12- 15 reps

-or-

Wide Grip Pull Ups to the back of neck 3 sets 8 -10 reps

Dave's Personal Shoulder Routine

Seated Behind The Neck Press 3 sets 8-10 reps

Upright Rows 3 sets 8-10 reps

Machine SIde Laterals 3 sets 8-10 reps

Dumbbell Shrugs 3 sets 8-12 reps

Dave's Personal Chest Routine

Flat Bench Barbell Press   3 sets of 8-12 reps

Incline Barbell or DB Press 3 sets of 8-12 reps

Seated Pec Deck Flyes   3 sets of 8-12 reps

Dumbbell Pullovers 3 sets of 8-12 reps

(you may use machine press for flat bench)

Dave's Personal Leg Routine

Barbell Squats   3 sets of 15-20 reps

Hack Squats   3 sets of 10- 12 reps

Leg Extensions   3 sets of 8-10 reps

Leg Curls   3 sets of 8-10 reps

(I like to start my first set only of squats off with a 25lb plate under each heel to really get more cuts on the tear drop in front of knees, and old fashioned floor hack squats are done in a similar fashion off the floor with barbell behind you lifting like a dead lift, but with heels elevated on block of wood or 25lb plates and the bar being grabbed from behind, kind of sit on the Olympic Bar with a 45lb on each side and then slowly stand up…wow it is a killer on the legs!)

Dave's Personal Calf Routine

Standing Machine Toe Raises 3 sets 15-20 reps

Toe presses on angled leg press machine 3 sets 12-15 reps

Stretch the calves between sets standing on your toe's

and pulling up for 10 reps between the weighted sets.

CHAPTER TWENTY-ONE

EXERCISES

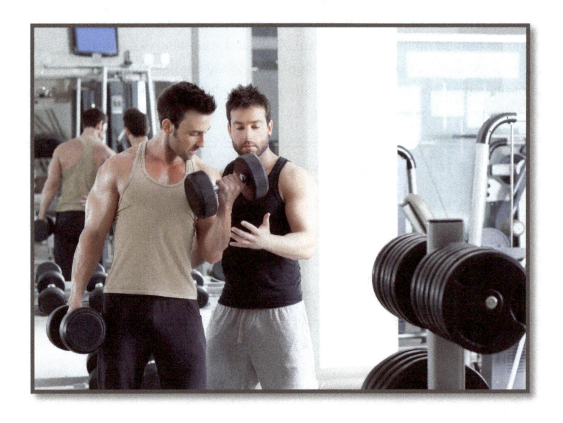

CHEST

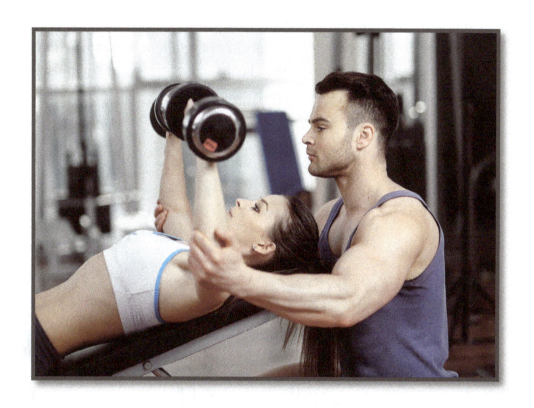

Barbell Bench Press

Starting Position: Lie on a flat bench with feet on the floor a little wider than shoulder width apart. Grab the bar with an underhand grip a little more than shoulder width.

Exercise: Raise the bar straight up and then lower the bar to the middle of your chest while breathing in, then press the weight back up while breathing out. Keep your back and hips flat on the bench; as it is best to not totally lock out when raising the weight back to the starting position since it keeps more tension on the muscle group. This completes one full repetition.

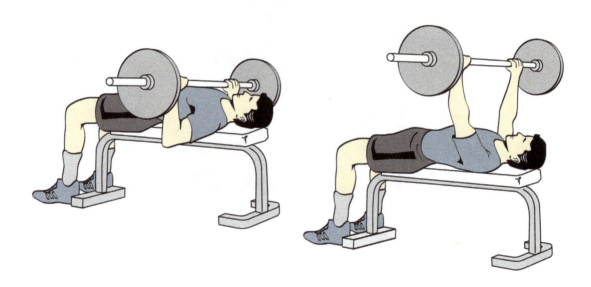

Machine Chest Press

Starting Position: Sit in machine and adjust seat so your chest is just above the handles.

Exercise: Grab the handles with a wide overhand grip and press the handles out until your arms are fully extended, then return to starting position. This completes one repetition.

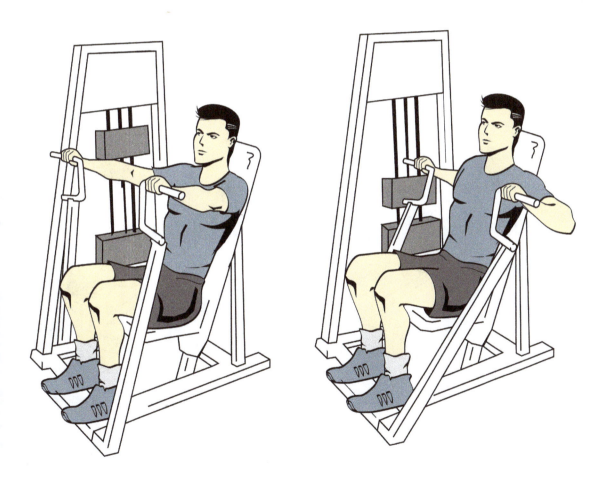

Decline Dumbbell Press

Starting Position: Lay on the bench, secure your feet under the holder, and rest your dumbbells on your thighs.

Exercise: Lower yourself down onto the bench and, holding the dumbbells in an overhand grip, bring them down to either side of your chest just above the shoulders. Keep your head flat on the bench. Press the dumbbells up with palms facing toward your feet — you will feel the stretch in the chest — then return to the starting position.

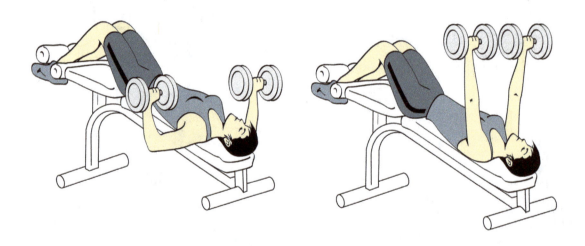

Dumbbell Bench Press

Starting Position: Lie on a bench holding a dumbbell in each hand just above your shoulders, palms facing forward toward your feet.

Exercise: Press the weights up while straightening your arms and bring the barbells together over the chest area. Then slowly lower them to the starting position once again. You will feel the stretch in the chest. This completes one repetition.

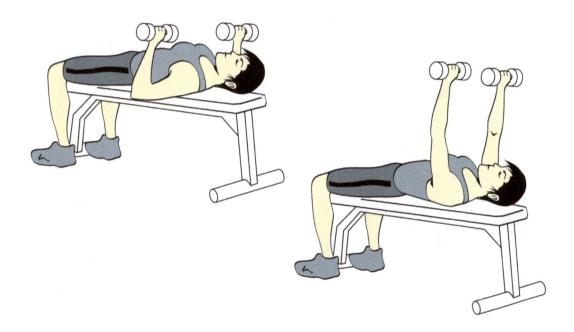

Incline Dumbbell Press

Starting Position: Sit on an incline bench. Grab a dumbbell in each hand and rest them on your thighs, then lean back while firmly pressing against the bench and firmly securing feet.

Exercise: Press the dumbbells up over your upper chest area as you straighten your arms, then inhale as you lower the weights back to the starting position. Keep the bench at a moderate angle and not too steep or you will work too much of the shoulder and not as much of the chest.

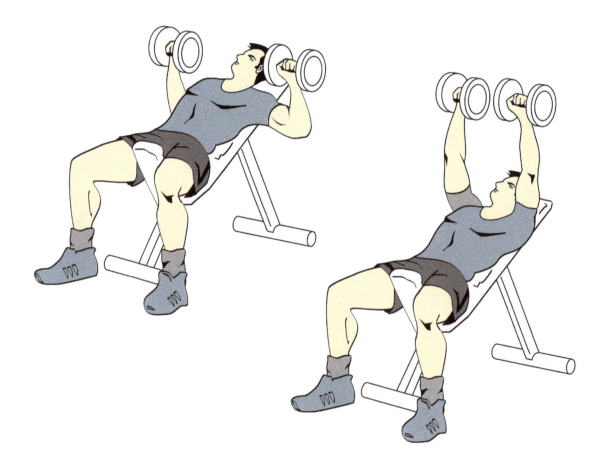

Dumbbell Pullover

Starting Position: Lie with your upper back across a flat bench. Lift a light dumbbell over your head and hold it above your face area.

Exercise: Slowly lower the dumbbell over your ear in an arc position while keeping your hips low and not raising them. Breathe deep while you're reaching a full stretch, then return the weight to the starting position while exhaling.

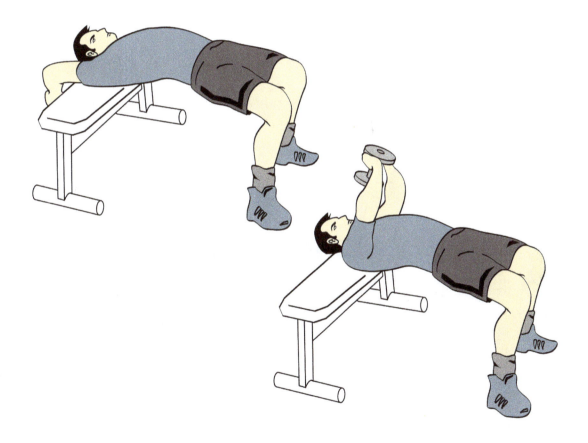

Dumbbell Flyes

Starting Position: Sit on a bench holding a dumbbell in each hand, then lie back onto the bench with the dumbbells at each side of your chest area.

Exercise: Press the dumbbells straight up and then have palms face each other. Now bring the dumbbells down in a slight arc out to the side of your chest area. Feel the stretch of the chest and remember this is like a bear hug motion. Keep the elbows slightly bent through the movement. Do not let your arms go lower than the bench.

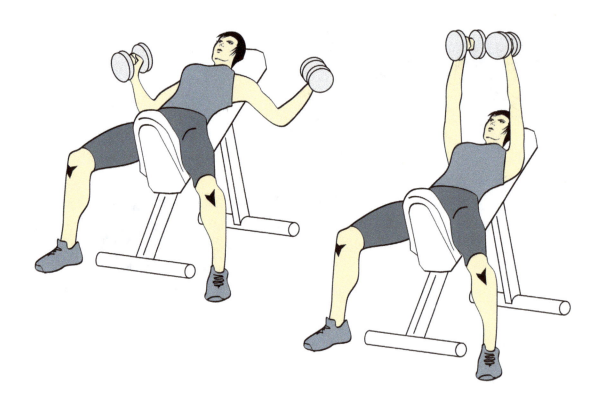

BACK

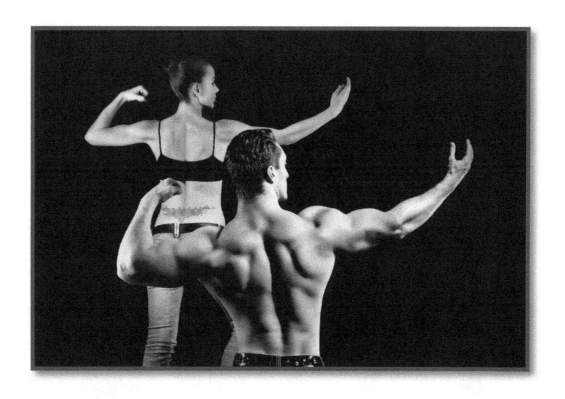

Wide-Grip Pulldowns

Starting Position: Sit on a pulldown machine. Put your knees firmly under the knee pads and grab the bar with a wider than shoulder grip.

Exercise: Pull the bar toward the top of your chest area. You may arch your back slightly while keeping firmly seated. Slowly let the bar up to the original starting position. That completes one repetition.

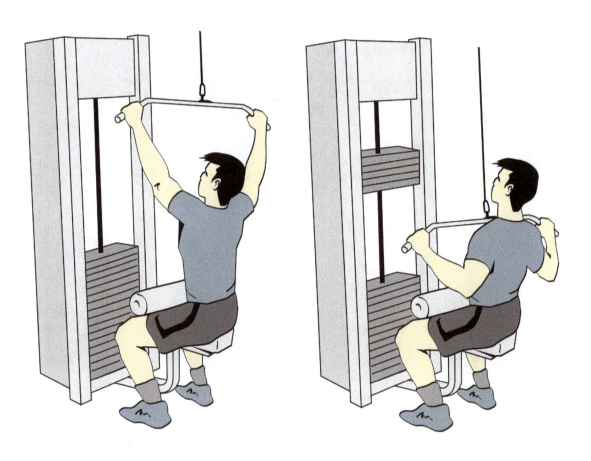

One Arm Dumbbell Row

Starting Position: Place your left foot flat on the floor and your right knee on a flat bench. Lean forward using your right hand for support on the bench. Your back should be straight parallel to the floor. Pick up a dumbbell with your left hand.

Exercise: Looking forward, pull the dumbbell up to the side of your chest, pulling your elbow as far back as you can, making the dumbbell parallel to your body. Slowly lower the dumbbell back to the starting position. Do not round your back. Squeeze your back muscles at the top of the movement. Do your set number of reps for this side and then switch sides and repeat.

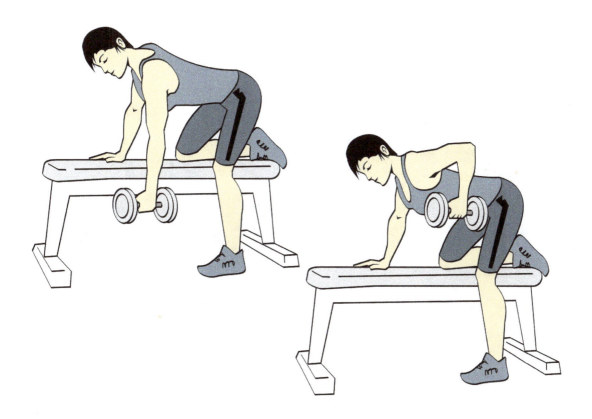

Bent Over Barbell Row

Starting Position: Grab a barbell resting on the floor with a shoulder with grip, palms facing you, then bend at the knee with your feet slightly wider than shoulder width apart.

Exercise: Looking forward, bend over with your back just about parallel to the floor. Lift the bar up toward you while you exhale. Do not move your torso. Keep your elbows tucked close to the body. Squeeze your back muscles at the top of this move. Inhale and lower the weight to your starting position. This completes one repetition.

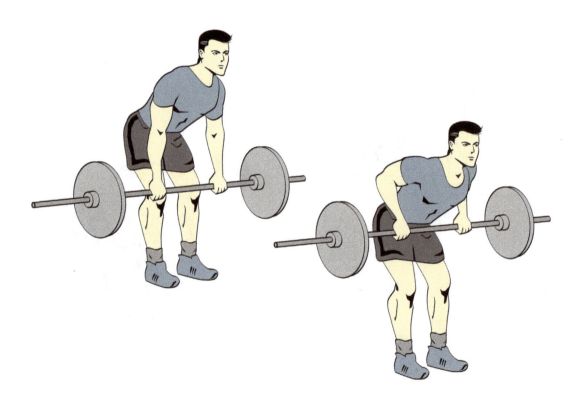

Seated Cable Row

Starting Position: Sit down on a cable row station. Connect a V-bar or pull bar to the cable. Plant your feet securely on the platforms, lean forward, and grab the bar with both hands.

Exercise: With your arms fully extended, pull back. Your chest will be slightly pushed out and your back slightly arched as you pull the cable toward your abdomen area, while keeping your torso stationary in position. Squeeze your back muscles and exhale as you bring the weight into you. Inhale as you return to the starting position.

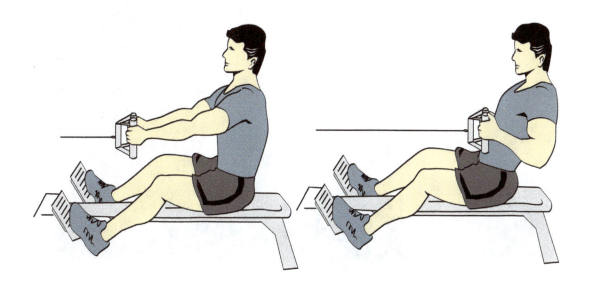

SHOULDERS

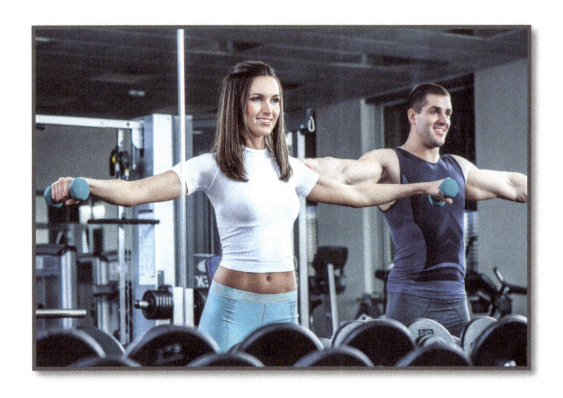

Seated Dumbbell Press

Starting Position: Sit on the end of a bench with your feet on the floor. Hold a dumbbell in each hand at shoulder height with your palms facing forward, away from you.

Exercise: Raise the dumbbells straight up, let the dumbbells almost touch above your head, then slowly return to the starting position. Exhale as you're raising the weight and inhale as you're returning to the starting position.

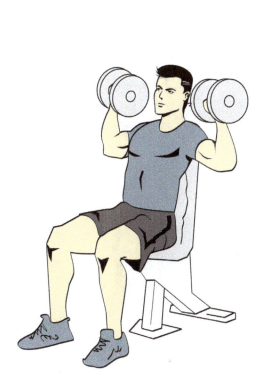
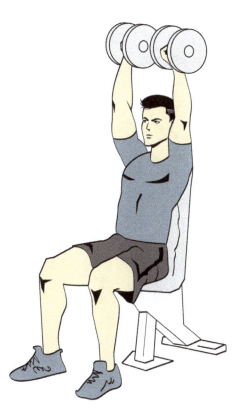

Side Lateral Raises

Starting Position: Standing straight up with your feet about shoulder width apart and your arms down at your sides, holding a dumbbell in each hand. Your palms will be facing in toward your body.

Exercise: Keep your arms straight and lift the dumbbells up and out to the sides of your body until they are at shoulder level just below the chin. Lower the weights back to the starting position. Remember to exhale as you raise the weight and inhale as you return the weight to the starting position.

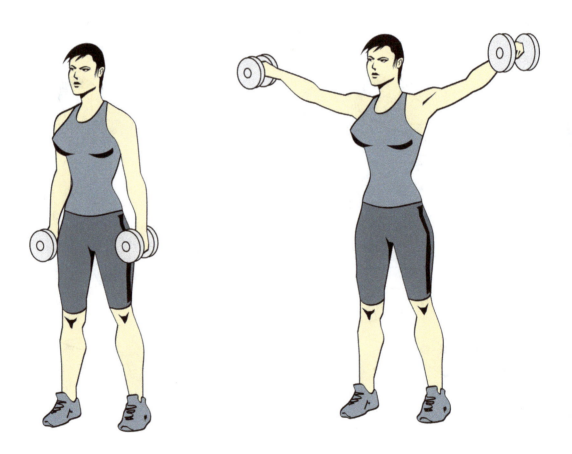

Upright Row

Starting Position: Stand straight up holding a barbell at your thighs with a grip less than shoulder width apart and your palms facing toward you.

Exercise: Lift the bar just below chin level using your shoulder strength and raise your elbows up and out to the sides while keeping the bar close to the body. Return the bar slowly to the starting position. This completes a full repetition. Exhale as you lift the bar and inhale as you return the bar to the starting position.

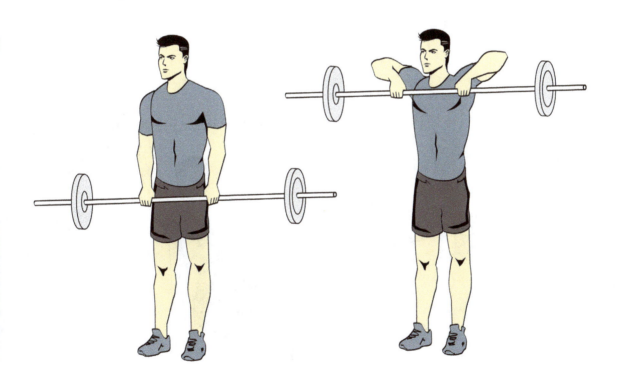

Seated Behind Neck Press

Starting Position: Sit down at a shoulder press rack with a back support and press your back firmly up against the straight up back pad. With both hands, reach up and grab the barbell with an overhand grip at shoulder width.

Exercise: Extend your arms and lift the bar off the rack. Inhale and lower the bar slowly behind your neck, then raise the bar back up to the starting position. This completes a full repetition. This exercise can also be done with dumbbells and standing if desired.

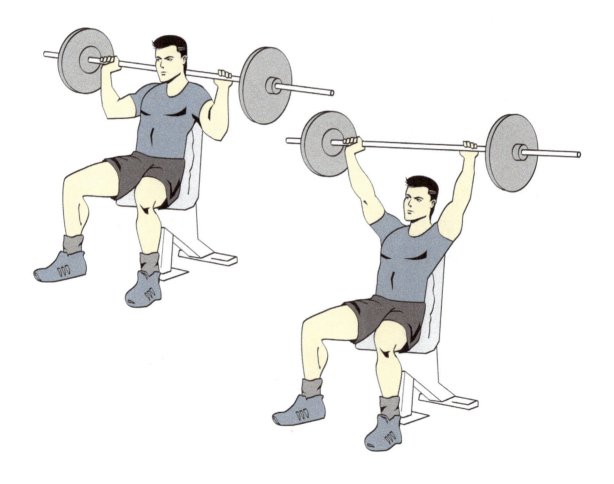

Dumbbell Shrug

Starting Position: Stand straight up with feet shoulder width apart and a dumbbell in each hand, palms facing in toward your body.

Exercise: Lift your shoulders in a shrugging motion raising the dumbbells, then relax the shoulders and return the dumbbells to the starting position.

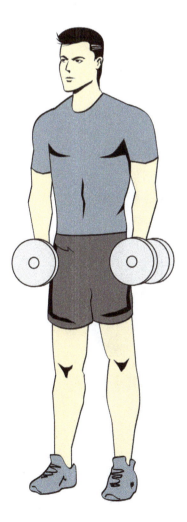
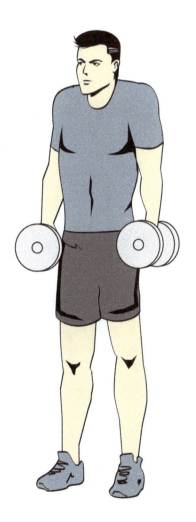

Front Dumbbell Raise

Starting Position: Grasp a pair of dumbbells and stand straight up with your hands facing the fronts of your thighs. Your feet should be about shoulder width apart.

Exercise: Looking straight ahead and moving just your arms, slowly raise the dumbbells one at a time to the height of your shoulder and then slowly lower the dumbbell back to the starting position and alternate between the right and left sides. First do the right and then the left. This will complete one repetition. Tighten your abdominals while doing this exercise as it will keep you from straining your back. Use a lighter weight for this exercise.

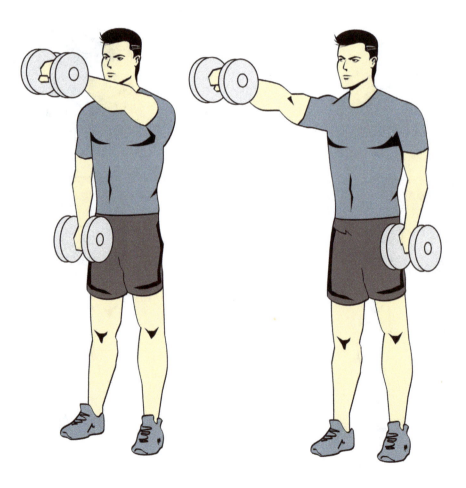

BICEPS

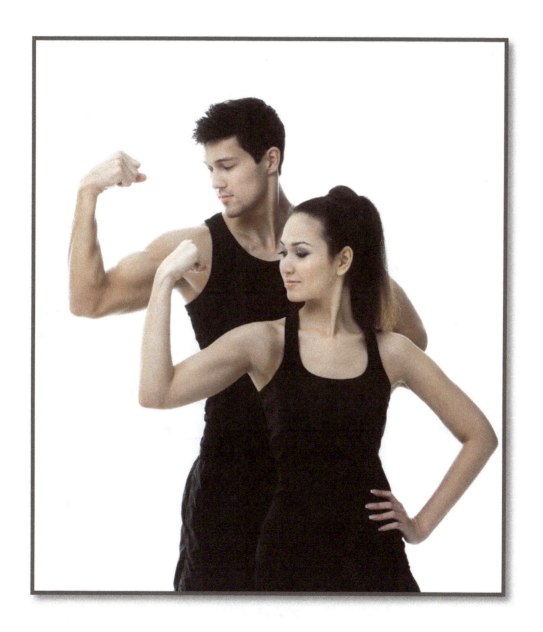

Incline Alternate Dumbbell Curls

Starting Position: Sit on an incline bench while holding a pair of dumbbells in each hand. Keep your shoulders square and pressed against bench and your chest elevated. Your hands will be hanging down to your sides, holding the dumbbells with palms facing forward.

Exercise: Slowly curl the right dumbbell up to shoulder height, squeezing the bicep muscle at the top of the movement and then slowly lower the weight until the arm is straight down again. Then repeat with the left arm, alternating between sides.

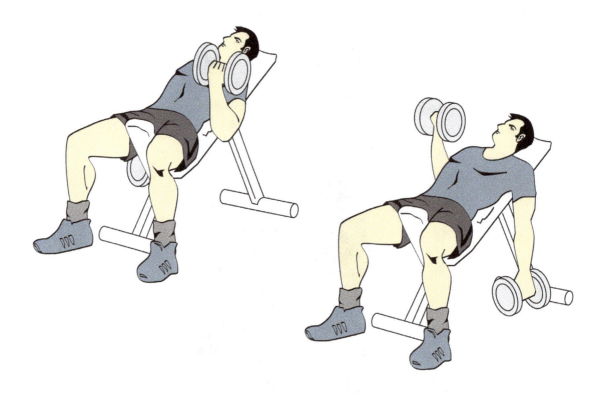

Standing Barbell Curls

Starting Position: Stand with feet shoulder width apart, holding a barbell at shoulder width with palms facing forward.

Exercise: Curl the weight up while standing straight up and not leaning back. Let your biceps do the work as you exhale. Tighten your abs to help you keep straight. Keep your upper arms close to your body while allowing your forearms to move. Once the bar is raised and the bicep is fully flexed and contracted, slowly move the bar back to the starting position as you inhale. This completes one repetition.

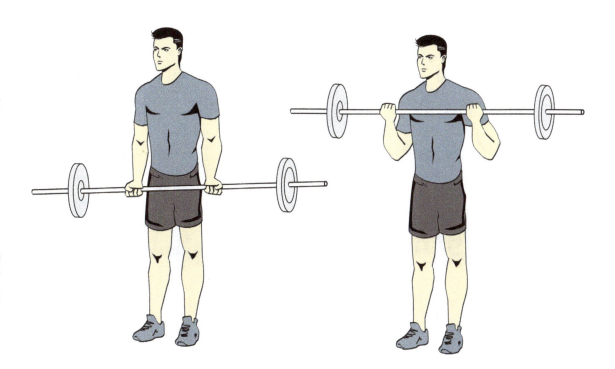

Standing Alternate Bicep Curl

Starting Position: Grab a dumbbell in each hand and stand straight up with feet firmly planted on the ground and abs tight.

Exercise: Curl the right dumbbell upward toward the shoulder and turn your wrist outward as you complete the full contraction of the bicep muscle and squeeze at the top of the movement, then slowly lower the dumbbell to the starting position and repeat with the left side. This will complete one repetition. This is an excellent bicep developer.

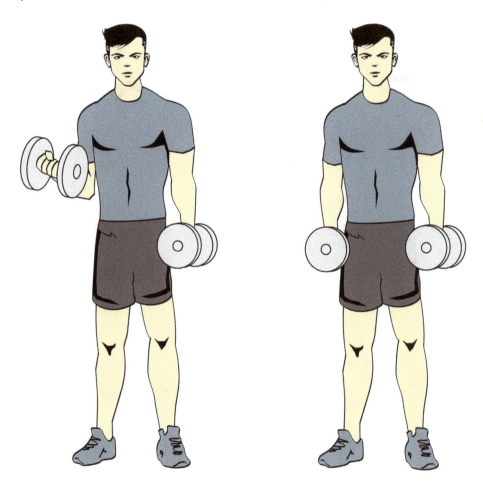

Preacher Curl

Starting Position: Sit at a preacher curl bench, free weight or machine. Adjust the seat so that is it the right height for your body. Rest your upper arms on the pad.

Exercise: Grab the bar with an underhand grip with both hands shoulder width apart. Curl the bar up toward your chin area and reach a full contraction of the bicep muscle, squeeze it at the top, then slowly return the weight to the starting position, keeping your hands on the bar the whole time until your repetitions are complete. This is an excellent bicep movement. (Developed by Larry Scott years ago, it is sometimes called the Scott Curl.)

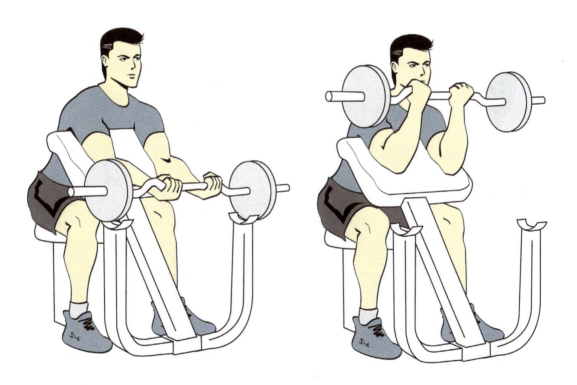

Concentration Curls

Starting Position: Sit on the edge of a flat bench with your legs spread in a V formation. and set a dumbbell between your feet. Grab onto the dumbbell with an underhand grip.

Exercise: Bend forward and, with your arm fully extended, hold the dumbbell. Place your other hand on your knee. With the dumbbell just above the floor and the back of the upper arm sitting on the inside of the thigh, curl the dumbbell up until the bicep in fully contracted, squeeze the bicep, then slowly return the weight to the starting position. Do your full set of repetitions and then repeat same procedure on the opposite side. This exercise is great for getting a peak in the bicep.

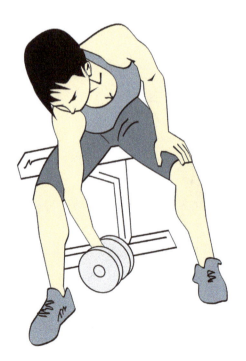
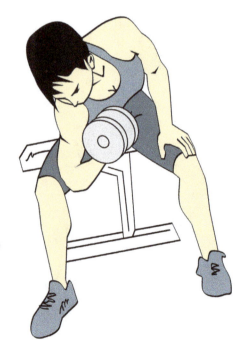

TRICEPS

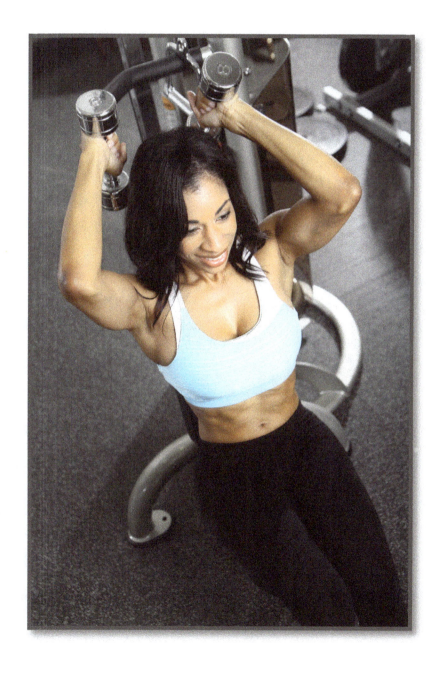

Tricep Pushdown

Starting Position: Using a cable machine, take a less than shoulder width grip, palms down. Feet should be shoulder width apart and your forearms should be at a parallel level to the floor as it holds the bar in the starting position. Bend slightly at the knees.

Exercise: Push the bar down, keeping your elbows close to the body as the bar moves toward the legs and the arms are straight out with the elbows in a locked position. Squeeze the triceps, then slowly return to the starting position.

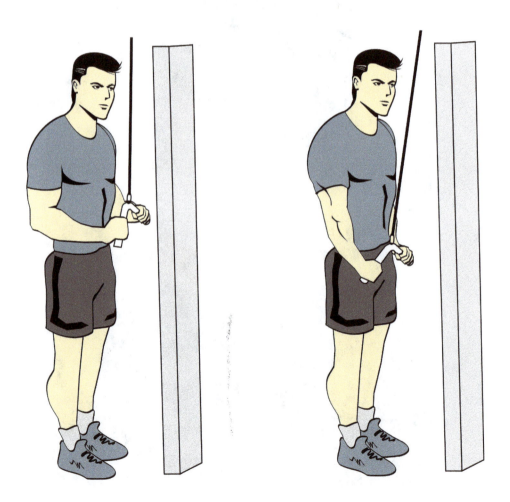

Tricep Kickback

Starting Position: Place your left knee on a bench and support your body with your left hand down on the front of the bench. With your right hand, pick up a light dumbbell.

Exercise: Holding the dumbbell, now raise it up to be in line with your body, keeping the elbow close to your side. Now, extend your arm and push the dumbbell back into a kick motion, squeezing the tricep at shoulder level. Slowly lower the weight and perform the desired repetitions, then repeat on the opposite side of the body. This is a good exercise to firm up the triceps and upper arm area.

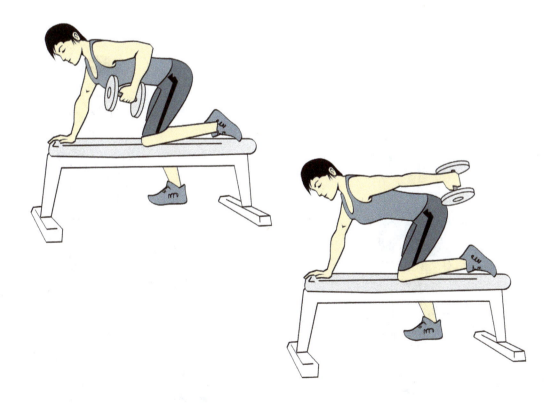

Seated Tricep Extension

Starting Position: Sit on the edge of a bench and grab a dumbbell at one end. Hold the dumbbell overhead with your arms fully extended and palms up.

Exercise: Keeping the elbows close to the head, bend your arms, slowly lowering the dumbbell behind your head. Your elbows should be pointed straight up as you lower the weight until you feel the full stretch in the triceps. Slowly return to the starting position with the dumbbell over your head and arms locked out. This completes one repetition.

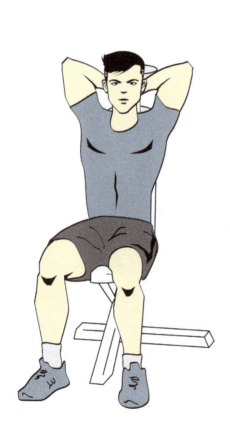 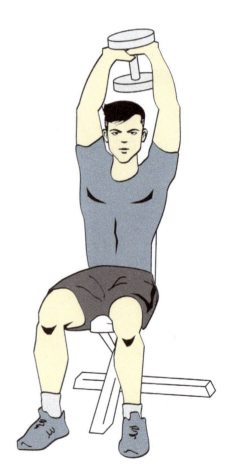

LEGS

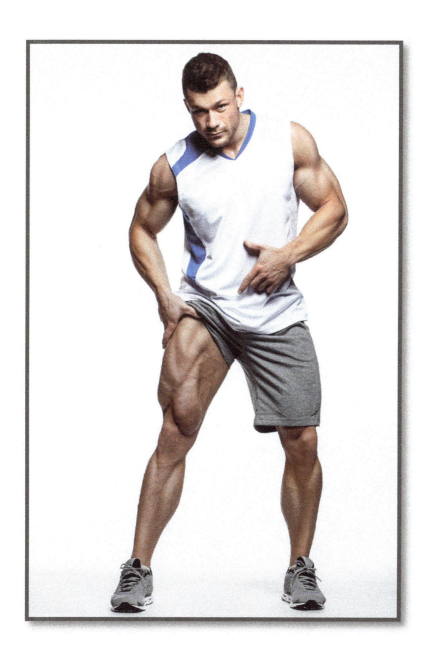

Leg Extensions

Starting Position: Sit down on a leg extension machine and place your ankles under the pads. Adjust the machine to fit your body. Grab hold of the handles on the side of the seat to help keep your body firmly in place.

Exercise: Straighten your legs out into a full extension, lifting with your quads until your knees are straight. Slowly lower the weight all the way down, keeping your hips on the seat. This completes a full repetition.

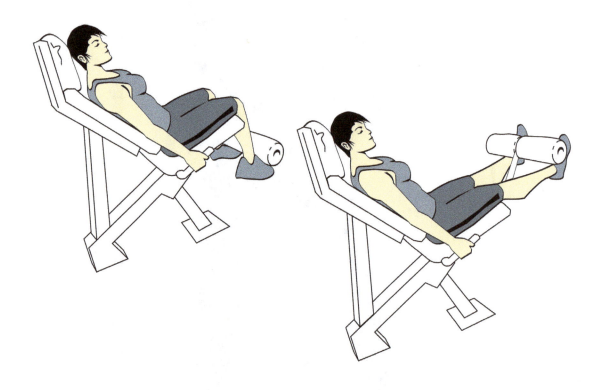

Leg Press

Starting Position: Sit down and position yourself onto the seat of the leg press machine. Place your feet, shoulder width apart, on the platform in front of you with the feet slightly pointed out.

Exercise: Release the safety handles while holding the weight up with your feet, then slowly lower the weight all the way down until your quads touch your stomach area as you inhale. Then push from your heels and return the weight to the starting position as you exhale, without fully locking out the knees at the top.

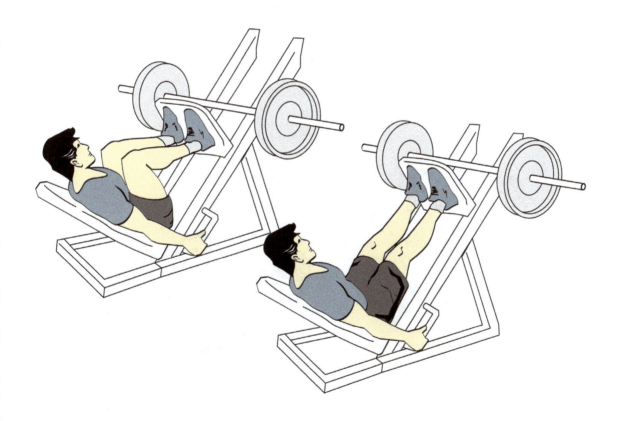

Barbell Squats

Starting Position: Stand in a squat rack with the barbell racked at about upper chest height. Get up under the bar and position your grip, palms forward wider than shoulder width and your feet at shoulder width, just slightly pointed out.

Exercise: Rest the bar on your upper shoulders and not on your neck. Lift the weight off the rack and lower your hips straight down until your thighs are parallel to the floor. Keep your chin up and do not bend forward. Once in the bottom position, then press the weight up with your heels to drive the weight up. Do not push with your upper body, just use your legs. Keep your abs tight. Inhale as you lower the weight and exhale on your way up. This is the best exercise for building great legs, but it is also the hardest. Start slow with light weight and good form, then work your way up into heavier weight or higher reps, depending on what your goal is.

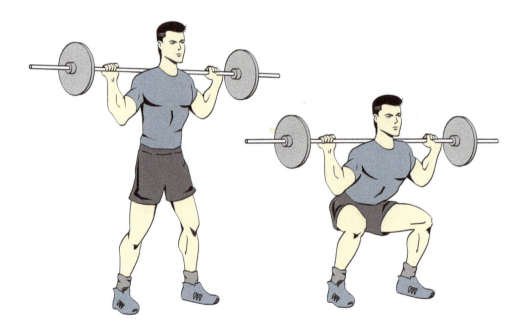

Dumbbell Lunges

Starting Position: Stand, holding a dumbbell in each hand, with your feet about eight inches apart and toes pointed forward. Keep your back straight and your chin up.

Exercise: Take a long step forward with your right foot, while bending your knees. Lower your body until your left knee is just above the floor. Push with your right leg, which will raise you back to the starting position. This completes one repetition. Do your target amount of reps and then switch sides.

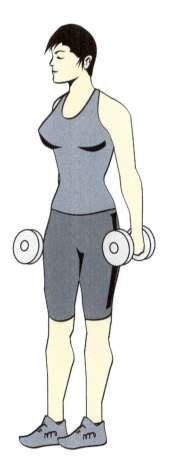
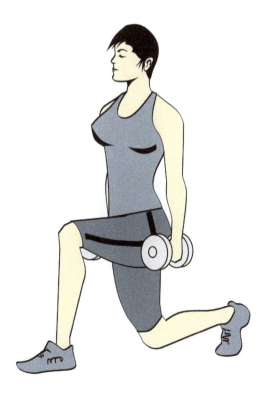

Dumbbell Squat/Deadlift

Starting Position: Standing up straight with your feet wider than shoulder width, place a dumbbell on the floor between your legs. Grab the top of the dumbbell with both hands and slowly stand straight up with your chin up and back straight.

Exercise: Slowly lower the weight in front of you until it almost touches the floor. Then return to the starting position while feeling it working your hamstrings, glutes, quadriceps, and lower back. Keep your abs tight during the movement to strengthen your torso.

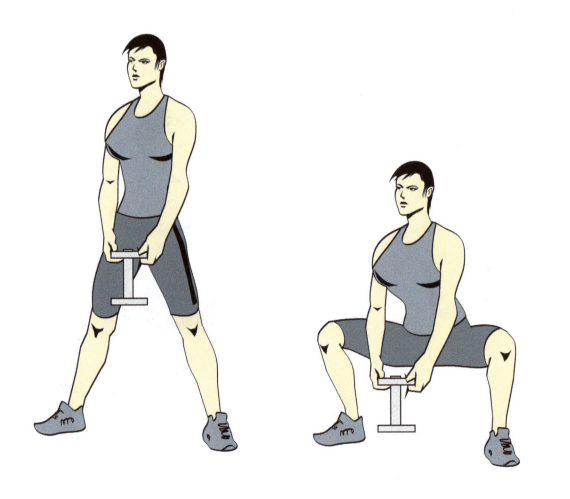

Lying Leg Curls

Starting Position: Lie face down on a leg curl machine and adjust the pads so they are on the back of your ankles. Grab onto the handles to secure your position.

Exercise: Slowly curl your legs up and bring your feet as close to your hamstrings as possible. Get a full range of motion and contract the hamstrings and glutes, squeezing the muscle at the top of the movement. Keep your body flat on the bench. This completes a full repetition.

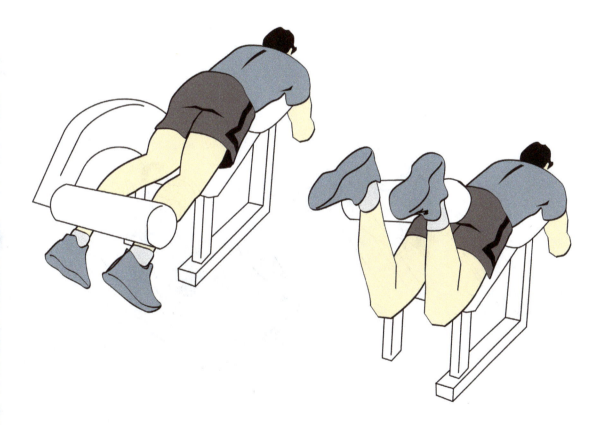

Machine Hack Squat

Starting Position: Step into the Hack Machine and place your back flat up against the back pad, placing your shoulders under the pads. Place your feet on the platform with your heels about eight inches apart and your toes pointed slightly out. Straighten your legs and release the safety latch.

Exercise: Slowly bend your legs and lower down into a low squat type position. Do not extend your knees past your toes. Straighten your legs by pushing down with your heels and returning to the starting position. Inhale as you lower the weight and exhale as you return the weight to the top. This is a good exercise for over the knee development and the full muscles of the thigh. This completes one repetition.

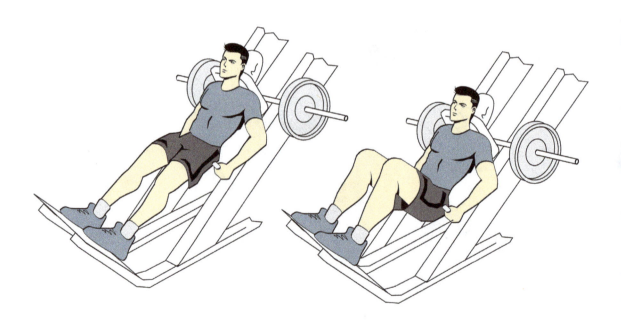

CALVES

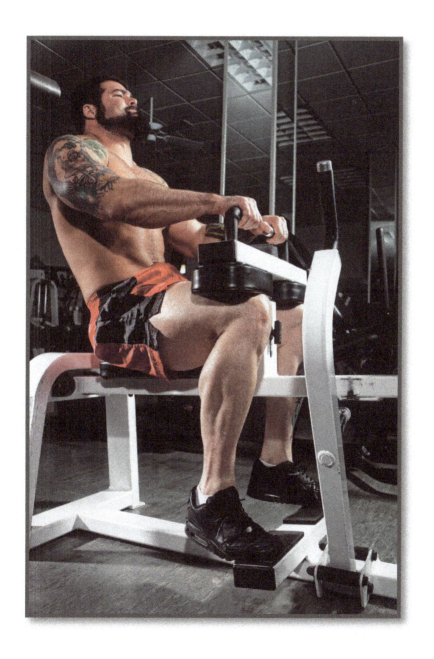

Standing Machine Calf Raises

Starting Position: Standing in the calf machine, adjust the height for your shoulders and position the balls of your feet on the platform and your shoulders under the pads.

Exercise: Do not bend your knees. Raise yourself up by lifting the calves onto the balls of your feet as far as you can, then hold and contract the calf muscle. Slowly lower your heels all the way down, keeping your shoulders and chin up while your hands hold onto the handles of the machine. Repeat for the desired amount of repetitions.

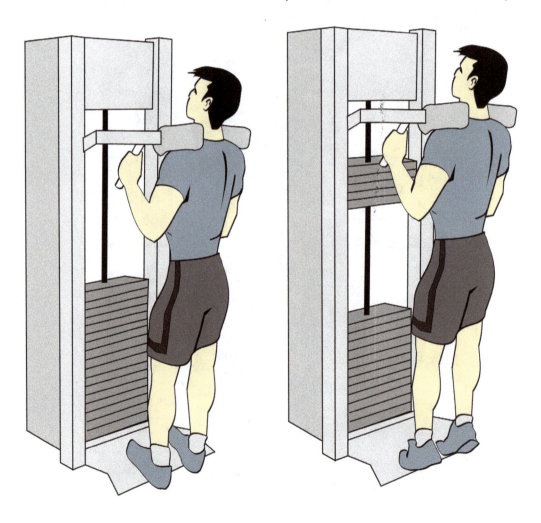

Seated Calf Raise

Starting Position: Sit on a seated calf raise machine with your lower thighs under the pads just above the knee and the balls of your feet on the platform. Keep as still as you can during the exercise, trying to only move the calves without rocking.

Exercise: Slowly raise up onto the balls of your feet and stretch as far up as possible, contracting the calf muscle, then slowly lower and repeat to the desired amount of repetitions.

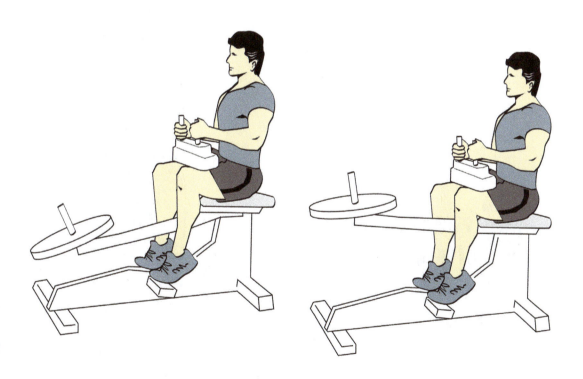

Dumbbell Calf Raise

Starting Position: Place two 25-lb weight plates, an exercise step, or 2x4 piece of wood in front of you that is about two inches in height. Grab a dumbbell in each hand and put your toes and balls of feet on the elevated surface you have chosen and put your heels on the floor.

Exercise: Lift your heels up as high as you can and push by the balls of your feet, contracting the calf muscle. Hold and squeeze it, then slowly lower to the starting position and repeat for the desired amount of repetitions.

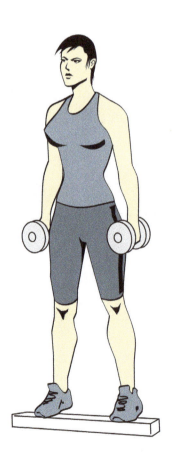
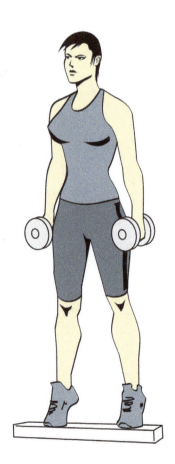

Toe Calf Presses

Starting Position: Sit in a leg press machine and place your toes at the bottom of the platform while holding onto the handles of the machine.

Exercise: Release the safety latch and, using only your toes, press and push the weight forward. Do not lower the weight toward you as you would in a leg press, but keep your knees locked and only press up with your toes until you fully contract the calf muscle, then relax toes, bringing them back to the starting position and repeat. Do not use as much weight as you would in a leg press, as this will be a much lighter weight in order to get a full contraction of the calves without involving the legs too much. Repeat until you reach your desired amount of repetitions.

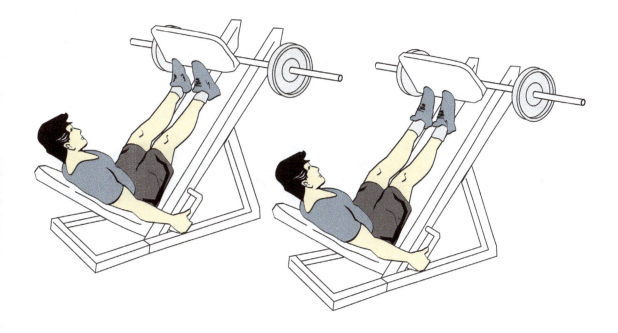

ABDOMINALS

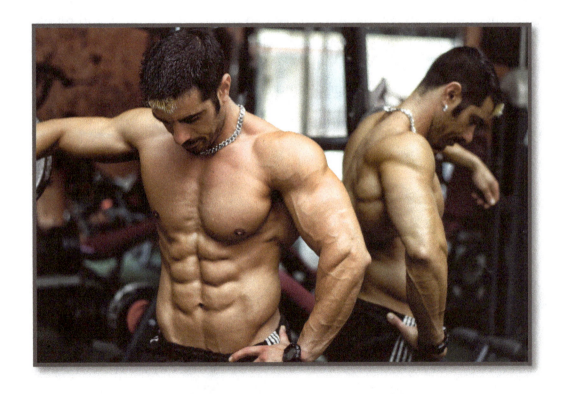

Floor Crunch

Starting Position: Lie flat on the floor, bringing your knees together and bent. With your feet flat on the floor, put your hands next to your head.

Exercise: Push your lower back down, keeping your knees stationary. Begin to gently lift your shoulders up as you push the abdominal back into the floor, squeezing your abs as you come up from the floor only a few inches. Do not put your hands behind your head, pulling your neck up — keep them at the sides of your head and let your abs do the work. This is a very good abdominal exercise as it is safer than a sit up and just as effective, if not even more effective.

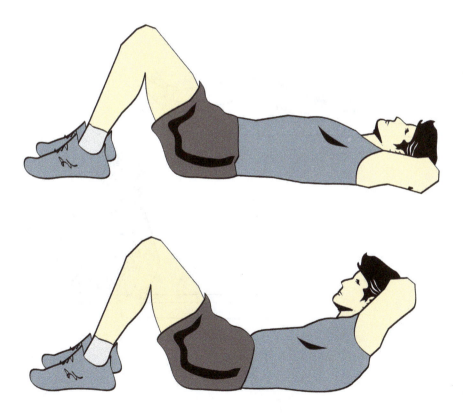

Bench Knee Pull-Ins

Starting Position: This is one of my favorites for abs. Sit on the end of a bench holding your legs out in front of you. Grab onto the sides of the bench to keep your body stable and securely in place as you lean back, holding your upper body at an angle.

Exercise: Pull your knees in toward you while moving your body toward your knees. Then return to the starting position and repeat. This is kind of like a combination sit up/crunch/leg raise all in one and gives you the benefits of all three combined. Complete the planned number of repetitions.

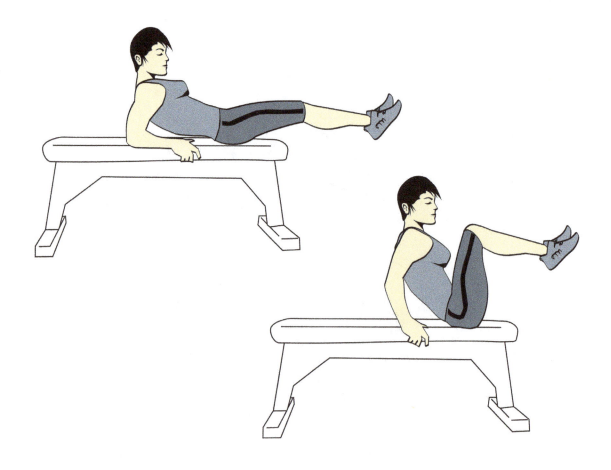

Machine Crunches

Starting Position: You can really benefit your abs by doing these machine crunches. Keep your back out of it and let your abs do the work. Sit in the abdominal machine and adjust the seat to your body. Put your feet under the foot pads and your elbows and triceps onto the arms pads as you grab hold of the hand grips.

Exercise: Slowly bring your upper body down into a crunch position and lift your knees up toward you, squeezing your abdominal muscles throughout the exercise. If your back, shoulders and arms are involved too much, then lower the weight. Let your abs do the work.

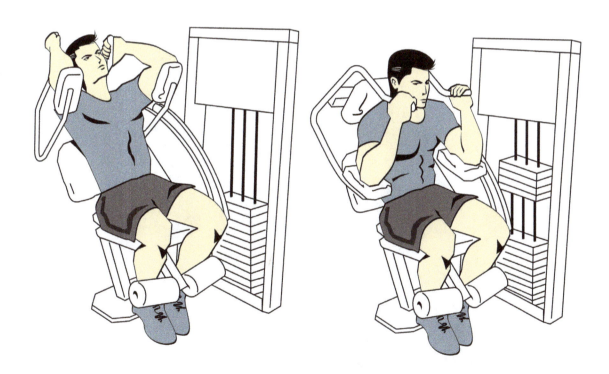

Side Bends with Broomstick

Starting Position: Stand with your feet shoulder width apart, chin up, and eyes looking forward. Place a broomstick handle behind your neck, resting on your upper shoulder area.

Exercise: Bend at the waist while holding onto the broomstick. Bring it down to your right side as far as you can, crunching the love handle area, then return to the starting position and do your left side. This completes one repetition.

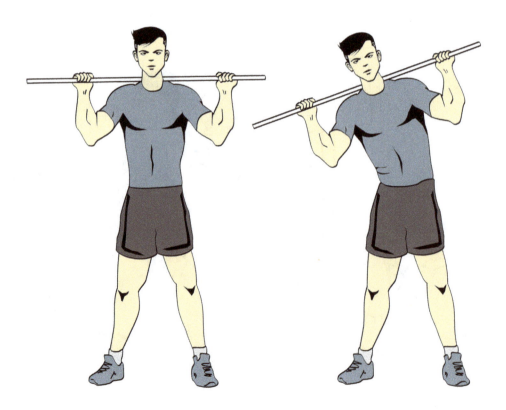

Side Twists with a Broomstick

Starting Position: Standing straight up with your feet shoulder width apart, or with your body seated at the edge of a bench, take a broomstick and place it behind the neck, resting on the top of the shoulder area. This will work the spare tire around the waist and tighten things up.

Exercise: Twist to the right, then to the left. That completes one repetition. Continue for your desired amount of repetitions. This will work the external oblique, the sides, intercostals and lower back. It's so simple it can even be done at home and combine with the side bends and crunches for a good home routine.

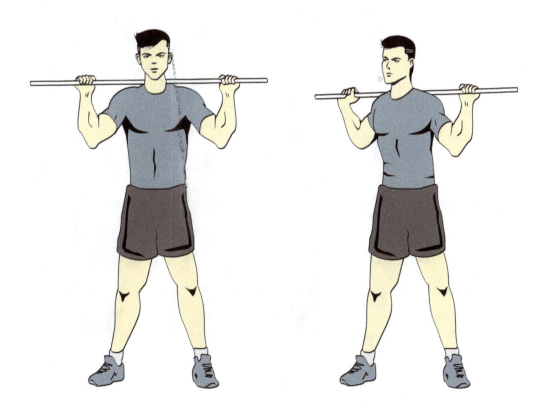

CHAPTER TWENTY-TWO
CARDIOVASCULAR EXERCISE

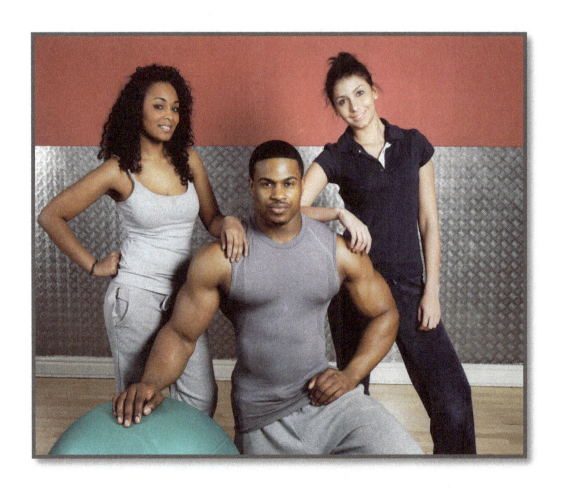

CHAPTER TWENTY-TWO
CARDIOVASCULAR EXERCISE

Before we get into in-depth talk about your cardio routines, let's look at a few other topics about your health.

What is Your Heart Rate?

Your heart rate (or pulse) is the number of times your heart beats per minute and it's also good to know what your resting heart rate is; in other words, what your heart is beating when you are at rest.

Okay, so first of all, your resting heart rate should be between 60 and 90 beats per minute. Now, this may be on the slower side if you're fit or have genetics that make you more apt to a lower rate. Now, on the other hand, it may also be faster if you're nervous or have consumed a large amount of caffeine, or are on medications or have high stress levels.

After approximately six to eight weeks of consistent exercise, your resting heart rate will usually drop. This will actually mean that your heart is doing a better job and has become more efficient. It may actually need to beat only 80 times per minute to pump the same amount of blood than it used to pump with 90 beats. This will save wear and tear on your heart makes so much sense when you think about it. It's just like any type of mechanical device. The more it's used, the sooner it will wear out and this is why preventative maintenance on our bodies is so very important.

If you would like to take your pulse, then here's how:

Rest your middle finger and index fingertips lightly on your opposite wrist, directly below the base of your thumb. If you can find the faint bluish line of your radial artery then place your fingertips there. It's within the same area below the base of the thumb.

Count the beats for one minute and there you have it.

What is Your Blood Pressure?

Blood pressure equals a measurement of how open your blood vessels are. If your numbers are low then that means your heart doesn't have to work very hard to pump the blood through your blood vessels. Your blood pressure should read 120 / 80 or below. A little variance is okay. However, if your blood pressure is higher than 145 / 95 then it would be considered on the high side. As your heart ejects blood, the bottom number measures pressure when your heart relaxes and prepares for the next pump. If your blood pressure is high, I recommend two products that my customers have had excellent results with. The first is called "Blood Pressure Factors" from Michaels and the second is "Flax Seed Oil," High Lignans, put out by Barleans. Take one or two tablespoons per day of the liquid for best results and the two products are all natural and may be used together.

The most popular way and most frequently used way over the years to determine one's maximum heart rate for men, is for a man to subtract his age from 220 and for women to subtract their age from 226. This formula will give you an approximate answer, but you should realize that it can actually vary ten to fifteen beats either way, but for the most part it has proven close to accurate in many that have used this method. This method is used primarily for activities in which your feet touch the ground. For bicycling – subtract five beats from the final result and for swimming – subtract ten beats.

So in other words, to find out your maximum, find your heart rate zone calculating 50 percent and 85 percent of your maximum.

Example: 220 – 40 = 180

This is his estimated heart rate.

180 x .50 = 90

This is the low end of his target zone. Now if his heart beats less than 90 times per minute, then he would know that he's not working out hard enough.

180 x .85 = 153

Now this is the high end of his target zone. If his heart beats faster than 153 beats per minute, then this tells him he needs to slow down!

Now with all exercise there is a warm up and a cool down period for which cardio is the favored exercise.

A warm up is considered approximately ten minutes of a very easy pace to get the body moving and warmed up, bringing it into the exercise mode, this also helps to put you into the proper frame of mind for your routine.

Next would be your regular workout, followed by a cooling down period which would also be for approximately ten minutes on the life cycle or stair climber to cool your body down and ease out of your workout routine.

How Much Cardio Should You Do?

Three 30 minutes sessions on the life cycle, tread mill, stair climber, jogging or brisk walking consistently done for at least six weeks will show significant results, especially if done on an empty stomach first thing in the morning, which forces your body to burn your fat stores.

Following this on, say, Monday, Wednesday, Friday would be a great start. You can even begin with three 20 minute sessions your first two weeks to train yourself and ease your way into the routine and then your longer term goal would be to work up to 45 minute sessions three times for one week or even increase to four 30 minute sessions if time permits.

You will feel the extra energy after you're consistent and into your routine for a couple weeks. All that oxygen will be getting into your bloodstream and it will start to make you feel refreshed, less stressed, more alert, more aware of your diet and overall a lot happier.

Remember the benefits of cardio are far reaching. These include:

* Improved cholesterol levels.
* Increased growth hormone.
* Increased metabolic rate for FAT burning and caloric burning.
* Improves digestion
* Helps increase blood flow to the brain
* Reduces stress
* Builds the immune system

Now remember it's okay to get in a 20-minute cardio workout of high intensity. Don't feel like your cheating yourself by not spending an hour at the gym. Research has shown that a 20-minute high intensity cardio routine actually will increase your metabolic rate for a longer period of time than a 40-minute low intensity workout.

My personal favorite is to get three (3) 30-minute cardio sessions per week first thing in the morning and get it out of the way. You'll burn more fat this way, since you'll have an empty stomach and you will feel better all day. You can do these three sessions on the opposite day from your workouts.

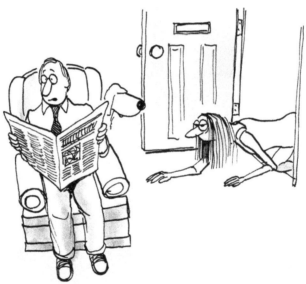

"How was aerobics class?"

Muscle Group Tolerance Chart

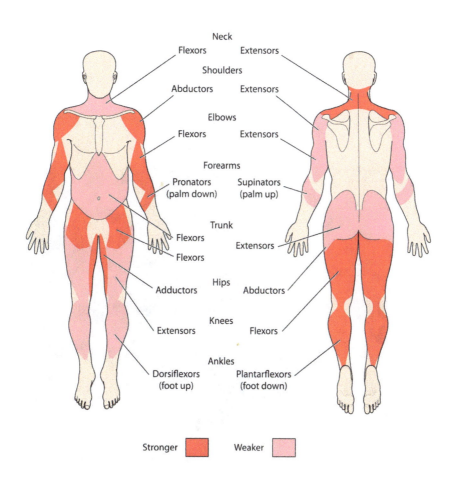

Neck
Flexors — Extensors

Shoulders
Abductors — Extensors

Elbows
Flexors — Extensors

Forearms
Pronators (palm down) — Supinators (palm up)

Trunk
Flexors — Extensors
Flexors

Hips
Adductors — Abductors

Knees
Extensors — Flexors

Ankles
Dorsiflexors (foot up) — Plantarflexors (foot down)

Stronger   Weaker

CHAPTER TWENTY-THREE
STRETCHING

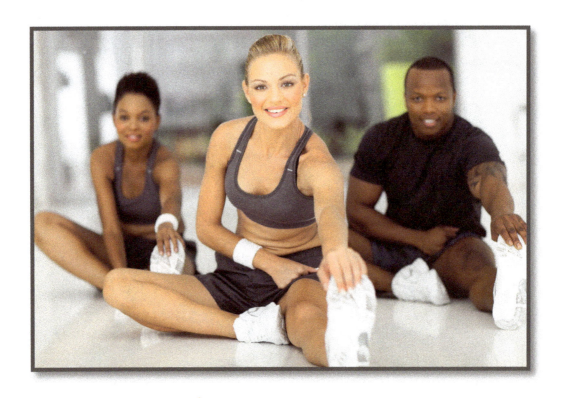

Hamstring Stretch

Sitting on the floor, extend your right leg out and bend your left leg, placing your left foot against the right inner thigh. Lean forward and reach for your ankle, trying to touch your toe while not straining too much. You want to be gently stretching out the area and should feel a slight pull in the hamstring. This completes one rep. Perform the planned number of repetitions for the set and then switch sides.

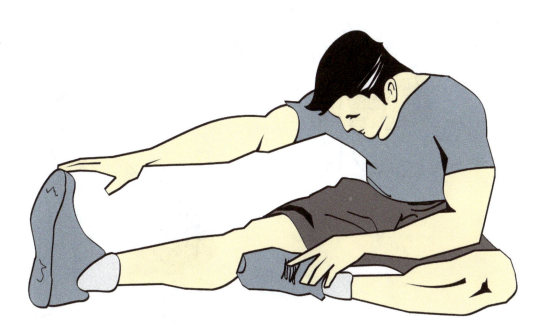

Cat Back Stretch

Kneel on the floor with your hands and knees shoulder width apart and chin up while looking forward. Now tighten your abs, pulling them in, hunch your back up, and flex your spine. Feel the stretch and then return to the starting position.

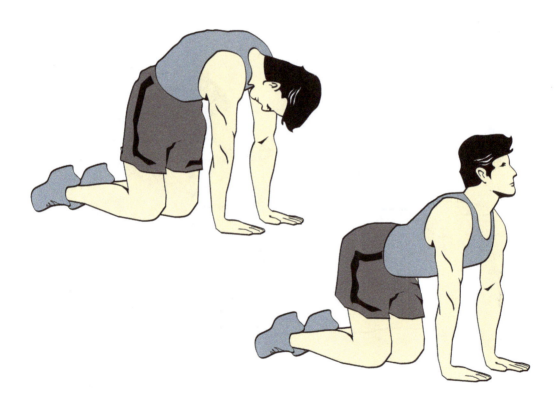

Leg and Calf Stretch

Facing a wall, place your hands on the wall with your arms fully extended. Lean against the wall, bending one leg forward and extending the other leg straight back. Dig the rear heel into the floor while bringing the hips forward just enough to feel a stretch. Perform the desired repetitions, then switch sides.

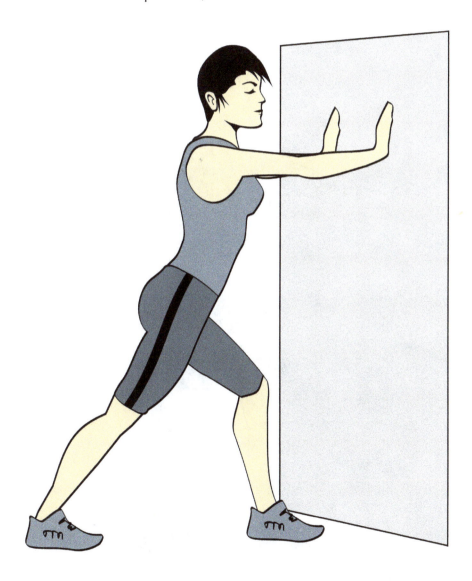

Chest Stretch

Standing straight with your chin up and looking forward, extend both your hands out in front of you so palms are touching in a pointing straight ahead grace form. Keeping your arms straight, now move the arms back as far as you can. Your palms will be facing forward now and you should feel a stretch in the chest area. Then return to the starting position. This completes one repetition.

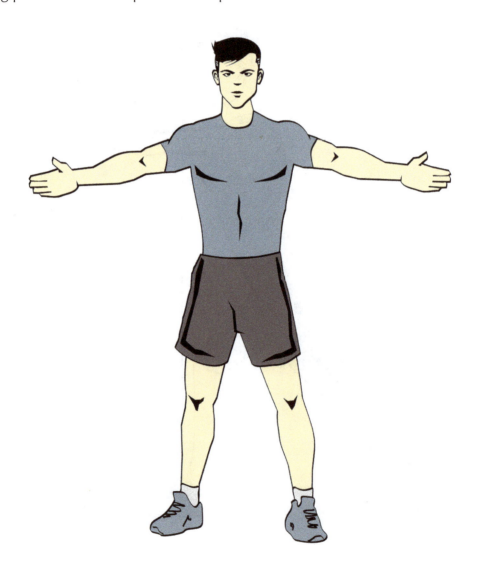

Lower Back Stretch

Lay down on the floor with your back flat and your legs extended in front of you, toes pointed towards the ceiling. Grab your right knee and gently pull it up to your chest area until you can feel a stretch in your lower back area. Return to the starting position and repeat with the left leg.

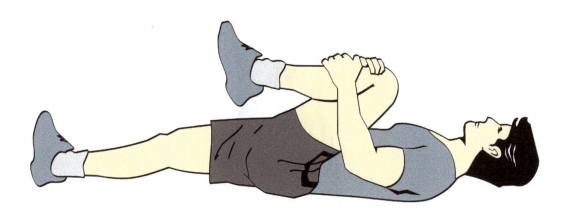

Shoulder Stretch

Standing straight up, bring your right arm across the front of your upper body and hold it with your left arm just above the elbow. Feel the stretch and then repeat with your left arm.

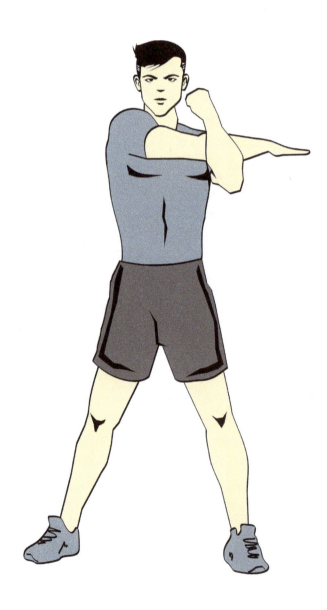

Abdominal Stretch

Lay face-down on the floor with your hands under your shoulders. Point your feet downward — this will lengthen the spine for the stretch. Slowly push your upper body up as far as you can, letting your hips rise slightly up off the floor. Raise your chin toward the ceiling, feel the stretch, then return to the starting position. This completes one repetition.

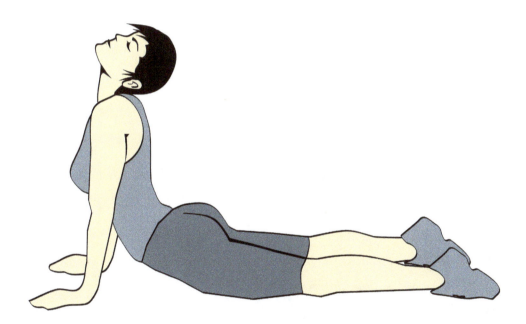

The following are some additional stretches you may want to try once you get used to the ones pictured.

Your body will most likely avoid injury if you are well stretched prior to training and stretch the muscles again after training. Make sure you gently stretch out the muscle groups and do not put too much tension on them.

This is in addition to your warm-up and cool down on the life cycle / treadmill or stair stepper.

Upper Back Stretch

<u>Purpose:</u> To stretch the hamstrings and lower back.

<u>Description:</u> Start in a standing position, legs straight and feet together. Bend over from the waist keeping legs and torso straight. Try to touch the ground on your ankles and do not rock. Hold for 30 seconds.

Inner Thigh Stretch

<u>Purpose:</u> To stretch the inner thighs.

<u>Description:</u> Sit on the floor or ground with your legs bent and the bottoms of your feet touching each other. Grasp your feet and pull them inward toward your groin as far as possible. Now relax the legs and drop your knees toward the floor, stretching the inner thighs. Press down on the knees for a deeper stretch. Hold for 30 seconds.

Calf Stretch

<u>Purpose:</u> To stretch calves and Achilles tendons.

<u>Description:</u> Stand arm's length away from a fixed object with your hands flat on the object at about shoulder height. Place your left leg forward and bend your knee slightly. Extend your right leg behind you, keeping it straight. Keep your right foot and heel flat on the ground and lean forward until you feel a stretch in your calf. Hold for 30 seconds. Switch legs and repeat.

Front of Thigh Stretch

<u>Purpose:</u> Stretches out the frontal thigh muscles that take on a lot of stress during leg training.

<u>Description:</u> Place your right hand on a chair for balance or fixed surface (wall) and grab your left foot behind you with your left hand and pull your heel gently towards your buttocks, repeat with other leg.

Shoulder Stretch

<u>Purpose:</u> Stretches out the shoulder muscles which is one of the easiest areas to incur an injury.

<u>Description:</u> Stand with your knees slightly bent and raise your right arm in front of you to shoulder height. Grab your right arm with your left hand, and pull your right arm across your body. Repeat with your other side.

Neck Stretch

<u>Purpose:</u> To stretch the neck muscles which will help avoid injury.

<u>Description:</u> Stand with your feet shoulder width apart, knees slightly bent, drop your head forward slowly stretching the muscles in the back of your neck then life head back up, placing hands behind back, take left wrist in right hand, drop your head to your opposite shoulder and pull gently down stretching.

A Foundation of Spiritual Fitness

A brilliant man once created modern mechanical technologies
that were often awed by many. And he thought he was happy,
but still felt empty. Then the brilliant man created tall skyscrapers.
And they too were awed by many. And he thought now he could
be happy, but he still felt empty. This same man built a huge city
in which his castle was the centerpiece and, oh, how it was awed
by many. And he thought now he could be very happy and
want for nothing — but he still felt empty. And then a great
hurricane came and destroyed the city he had developed and all his
modern mechanical technologies he had founded. The man then
wept and fell to his knees and he cried out to God and prayed for
the storm to stop and for his life to be spared. And then the rains
and winds stopped, the clouds opened, and the sun began to shine.
The man rose from his knees and looked toward Heaven as a tear
of joy came from his eye. He then said, I have nothing material
left, but I have found a relationship with God. I have remembered
my creator that I so often had forgotten. The man went on to
rebuild the city and this time all of his awesome creations were
built on a solid foundation that included GOD.

Now The Man Felt Happy!

Remember to always build your body from the inside out.

Make God your foundation to place everything else on.

"Potential Fitness"

We all have God given talents

and it's in recognizing these talents

and pursuing your gifts

that divides the achievers

from the non-achievers.

Make no mistake about it,

YOU are Special and

YOU have "Great Potential".

Now it's time to take your "Specialty" and

PRACTICE IT,

PERFECT IT,

BE CONSISTENT IN IT,

ENJOY IT,

BELIEVE IN IT,

OWN IT,

and You

WILL ACCOMPLISH IT!

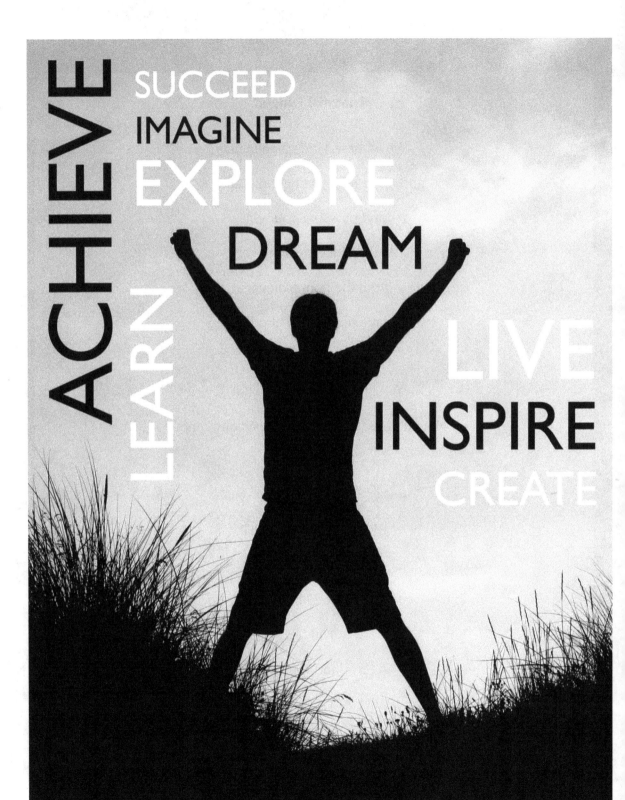

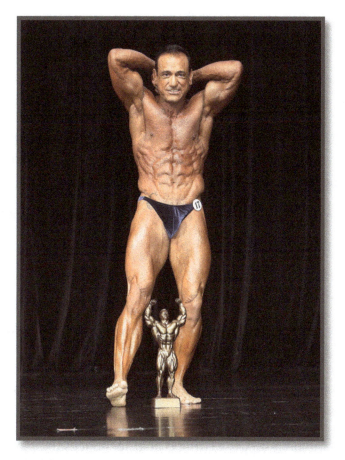

David Anthony Cucuzza
2015 NPC Florida State N.Q. Masters Class First Place
2014 NPC Seminole Classic Masters Overall Champion
2014 NPC Seminole Classic Master's 50+ First Place
2014 NPC JAX Physique Master's Class First Place

Good luck on your fitness journey and remember that owning your body and owning your faith equals the best formula for true fitness from the inside out.

www.nfmbody.com

www.naturesmarketorlando.com

REFERENCES:

American Heart Association, Nutrition Committee, good and bad fats, circulation, 2006; vol 114: pp 82-96.

Antonio J. et al. The effects of Tribulus Terrestris on body composition and exercise performance in resistance-trained males. Internal Journal of Sports Nutrition and Exercise Metabolism 10(2):208-215, 2000.

Artificial Food Coloring Dangers, Science News, Posted May 9th, 2008. Http://www. Science-News. Org/artificial-food-coloring.

Balch, Phyllis, A., CNC, Balch, James, F, MD, Prescription for Nutritional Healing, 3rd Edition, Penguin Putnum, Inc.,2000.

Barefoot, Robert, R., Reich, Carl, J., The Calcium Factor, Deonna Enterprises Publication, November 1, 1992.

Beck S, Olek A, Walter J. Genomics to Epigenomics: A loftier view of life. National Biotechnol.1999, December;17(12):1144.

Biolo G. et al. An abundant supply of amino acids enhances the metabolic effect of exercise on muscle protein. American Journal of Physiology: Endrocrinology and Metabolism 273(1PT1):E122-E129,1997.

Bibra Toxicology Advice and Consulting, http://www.bibra-information.co.uk.

Buckel, Jane, RN, Phd. Clinical Aromatherapy: Essential oils in practice, Churchhill Livingstone Publishing,2003.

Burgio PA., A literature review of velvet antler: The global market, chemical composition, health benefits and factors affecting growth. Erik Research Council;1998.

Candeloro N. et al. Effects of prolonged administration of branch-chain amino acids on body composition and skeletal muscle in older men. Journal of Applied Physiology 86(1):29-39,1999.

Cathy Wong, ND, Alternative Medicine, remedies for high cholesterol, http://www.about.com September 2013.

D' Adamo, Peter Dr., Eat Right For Your Blood Type, http://www.dadamo.com.

Green Coffee Bean Extract, double blind study, University of Scranton, Scranton, PA.USA 2012

Goss RJ, Dear Antlers: Regeneration, function and evolution. Orlando, Florida: Academic Press,Inc.1988.

Harvard Medical School, Family Health Guide, The Benefits of taking Probiotics,

Harvard Health Publications, September 2005.

Journal of the American Medical Association, Human weight-loss study, The effects of Garcinia Cambogia extract in humans. November 11, 1998

Journal of Obesity: The use of Garcinia Cambogia extract as a weight-loss supplement. Garcinia Cambogia;The newest, fastest, fat-buster,11-5-2012, http://www.Doctoroz.com

Kritchevsky, D. Conjugated linoleic acid, nutrition bulletin 25(1):25-28,2000

Law AJ and Kever J. Effect of PH on the thermal denaturation of whey protein in milk.

Journal of Agriculture and Food Chemistry 48(3):672-679, 2000.

Lemon PWR. Do athletes need more dietary protein and amino acids? Internal Journal of Sports Nutrition 5:539-561,1995.

Leslie Bonci, Director of Sports Medicine, Eat Right For Your Blood Type, University of Pittsburgh Medical Center, Posted 4/18/2011.

Lifestyle Guide, Vitamins and Supplements;DHEA,2013 http://www.webmd.com

Mcleod, Kerry, The Scary Truth About Food Coloring, Science News, Sept. 2008 http://www.sheknows.com

Mijnhout, G. The Netherlands Journal Of Medicine, Alpha Lipoic Acid, April 2010; vol68: pp158-160.

Mozaffarian,D. New England Journal of Medicine, good and bad fats, April 13,2006; vol 354:pp1601-1613.

Muller, A., Rice, PJ., Ensley, HE.,et al. Plasma lipid changes after supplementation with Beta Glucan fiber from yeast. AM, CJ, Clinical Nutrition 1999;70:208-12.

National Academy for Health and Fitness, Professional Health, Fitness and Exercise Manuals, N.A.H.F 1998, 2002.

Reprod Biol Endocrinol 2009 Oct 27;120 D'aspartic acid.

Roberts, AJ, O'Brian ME, Subak-Shape G. Nutraceauticals: The Complete Encylopedia of Supplements, Herbs, Vitamins and Healing Foods. Perigee Press/Penguin Publishing Group,2001.

Rowbottom, DG, Keast, D., Morton, AR. The emerging role of L-glutamine as an indicator of exercise stress and overtraining. Sports medicine 21(2):80-97, 1996.

Sears, Al, M.D. Power of Healthy Living. Information on DNA provided by Al Sears, M.D., For more information or to sign up for a free subscription to the doctor's house call e-letter, please visit http://www.alsearsmd.com

Sahelian, Ray. IP-6 Inositol Hexaphosphate Supplement. http://www.raysahelian.com/ip-6.html

Stout, JA., et al. The effects of Creatine supplementation on anaerobic working capacity, Journal of strength and conditioning research 13:135-138, 1999.

The Catholic Bible, Personal Study Edition, Oxford University Press, 1995.

The Holy Bible, King JamesVersion, Thomas Nelson Publishers, 1972.

Time Magazine, Why your DNA isn't your destiny. January 18th, 2010 Issue. Time Magazine Publications. *Additional references available upon request on all content

Toxic Food Additives, top 50, Alliance for Sustainable Communities Lehigh Valley, Posted September 2012 by PKC. http://www.mphprogramslist.com/50-jawdrippingly-toxic-food-additives-to-avoid.

Van Marle, Aarsen, PN, Lind A. Van Weeren-Kamer J., Deglycyrrhizinised Liquorice and the renewal of rodent stomach epithelium, Eur J Pharmacol 1981.

What are the benefits of taking Colloidiol Silver? Health and Wellness report: Colloidiol Silver 2013 http://www.Livestrong.com

DISCLAIMER